STAGE 4
KIDNEY DISEASE
COOKBOOK FOR SENIORS

Healthy, Easy to Prepare Low Sodium and Potassium
Recipes for the Elderly

HILDA M. JACOBS

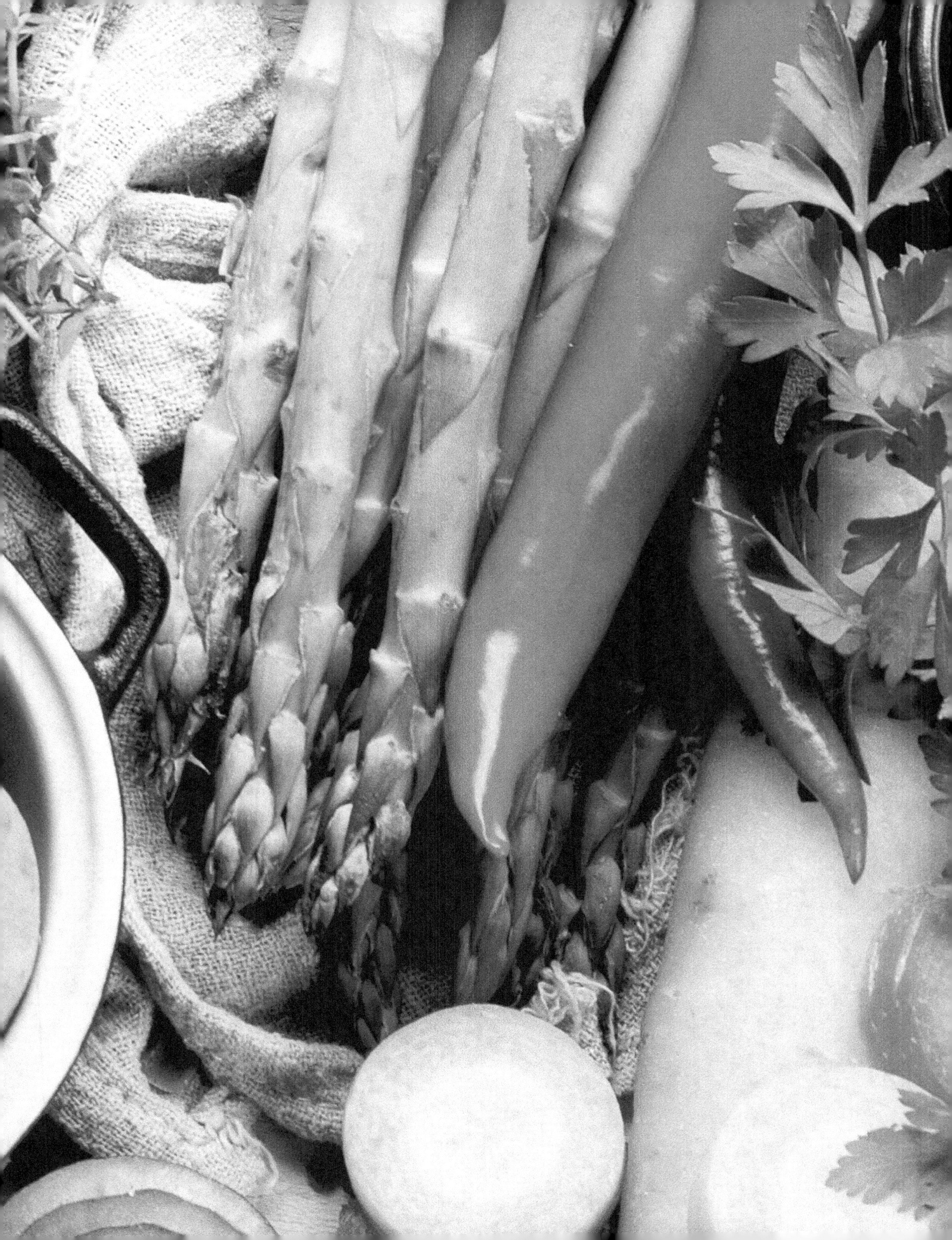

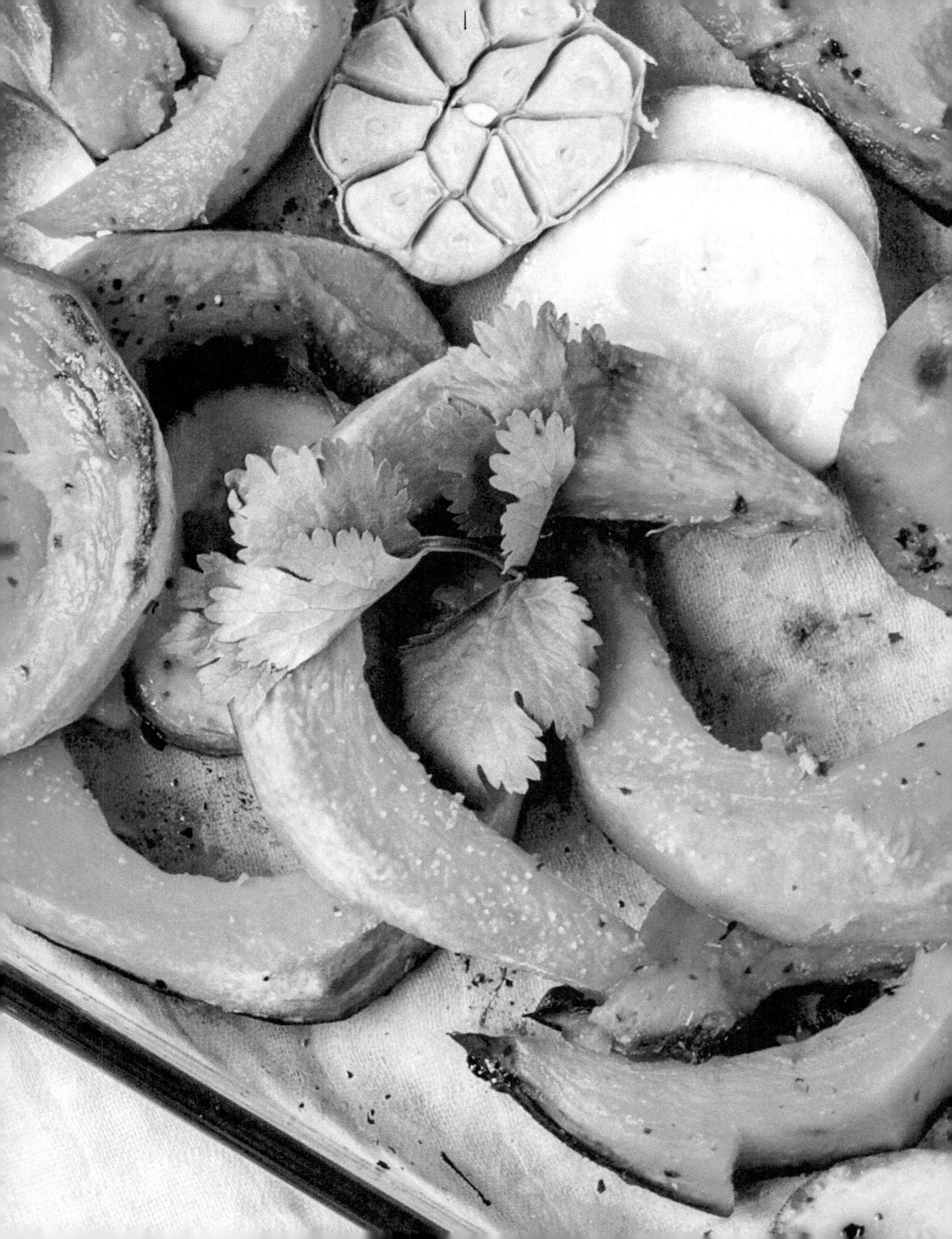

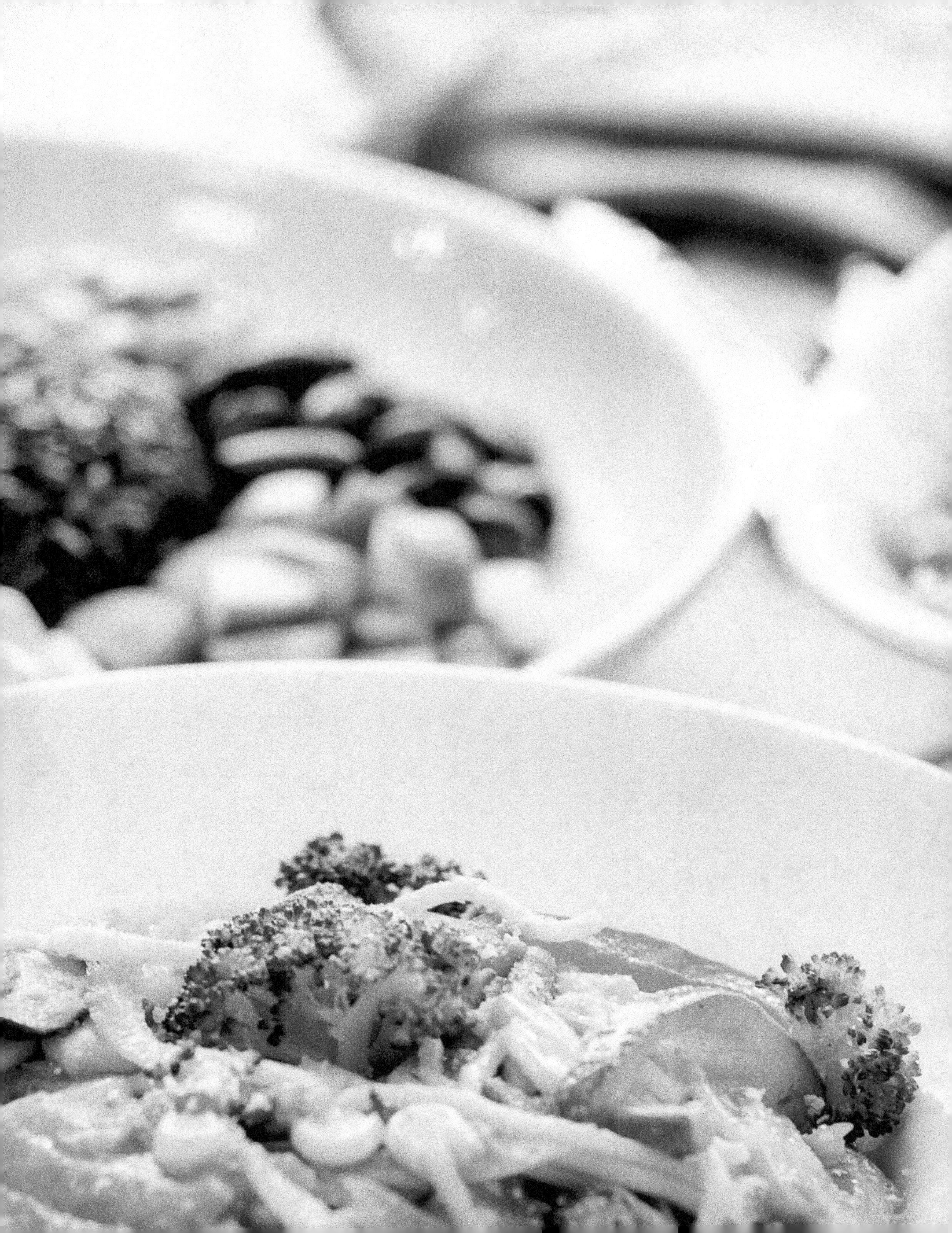

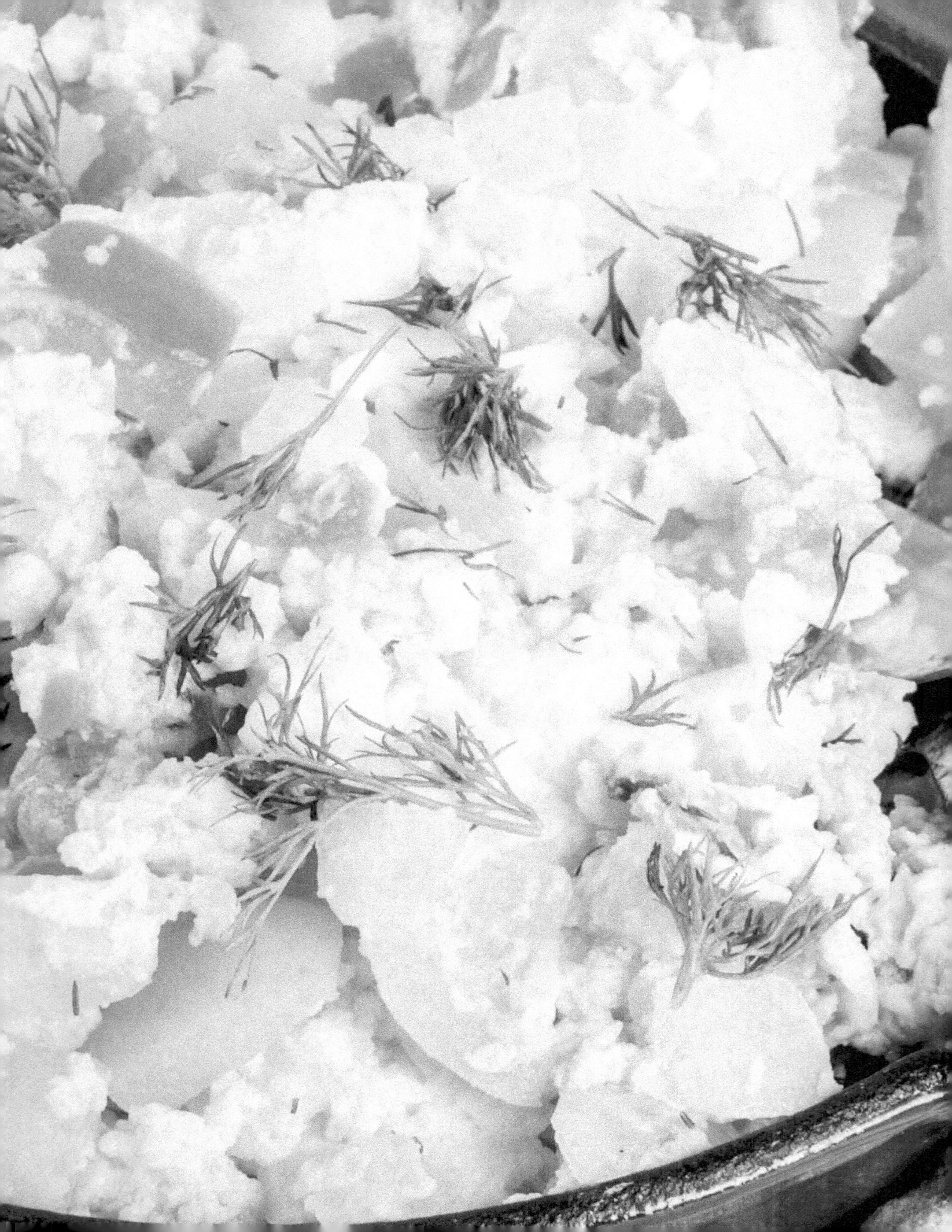

CONTENTS

INTRODUCTION 1

UNDERSTANDING STAGE 4 KIDNEY DISEASE...4

What Stage 4 Kidney Disease Really Means 4

Root Causes and Contributing Factors to Stage 4 4

Symptoms of Stage 4 5

NUTRITIONAL GUIDELINES FOR STAGE 4 CKD IN SENIORS 6

The Foundation of Disease Management in Stage 4 Kidney Disease..................6

Role of Proteins in Kidney Disease Management 7

Micromanagement of Micronutrients in Kidney Disease 9

Role Fluids in Kidney Disease 10

Role of Fiber and Antioxidants in Kidney Disease.......................................12

MEAL PLANNING AND PREPARATION..14

Creating a Kidney-Friendly Kitchen 14

Designing Your Meal Plan.........................16

Smart Shopping Strategies 17

Cooking Techniques and Tips 18

Eating Well Outside the Home.................20

BREAKFAST 22

Apple Puffs...22

Banana Oat Shake 22

Banana-Apple Smoothie 23

Berrylicious Smoothie...............................23

Blueberry Lemon Pound Cake 24

Chicken and Zucchini Quiche 24

Cranberry Ginger Apricot Chutney.............25

Fruit Crisp 26

Grilled Low-Salt Flatbread........................26

Love Your Kidneys Breakfast Cereal.........27

Peanut Butter Oatmeal..............................28

Pumpkin Pancakes...................................28

Pumpkin Cream Cheese Muffins................29

Turkey Bacon, Egg, and Cheese Deviled Eggs 30

Lemon-Blueberry Corn Muffins.................30

Blueberry Oatmeal...................................31

Blueberry Squares 32

Bran Breakfast Bars 32

LUNCH **34**

Apple Rice Salad.................................... 34

Baked Macaroni and Cheese 34

Baked Potato Soup 34

Beef Barley Soup 35

Canned Fish Tacos 35

Chicken and Corn Chowder 36

Chicken and Dumplings 36

Chicken N' Orange Salad Sandwich.......... 37

Chinese Chicken Salad............................. 38

Cider Cream Chicken 38

Cowboy Caviar Bean and Rice Salad 39

Creamy Tuna Twist................................. 39

Curry Chicken Salad 40

Fruity Chicken Salad............................... 40

Green Tomatoes with Goat Cheese........... 41

Grilled Vegetable Pasta Salad 41

Herb Breaded Chicken 42

Irish Baked Potato Soup.......................... 42

Kohlrabi Soup 43

Lemon Curry Chicken Salad 44

Lentil Meatballs or Patties........................ 44

DINNER **46**

Apple Almond Galette 46

Apple Caramel Crisp................................ 46

Apple Cranberry Walnut Salad 46

Apple Sage Stuffing 47

Birthday Popcorn 47

Bolognese with Rice Noodles 48

Bow-Tie Pasta Salad 48

Creamy Curry Rice & Apple Salad............ 49

Favorite Cranberry Salad 50

Grilled Vegetables................................... 50

Mexican Antojitos................................... 51

Moroccan Couscous 52

Apple Spice Cake 52

Roasted Asparagus and Wild Mushroom
Stew.. 53

Balsamic Marinated Mushrooms 54

Blueberry Lemon Pound Cake 54

Creamy Curry Rice & Apple Salad............ 55

Favorite Cranberry Salad 56

Gelatin Beet Salad................................... 57

Healthy Chicken Nuggets......................... 57

Grilled Vegetables with Herbed
Vinaigrette.. 58

Mexican Antojitos................................... 59

DESSERT **60**

Baked Shrimp Rolls 60

Barbecue Meatballs 60

Brie and Cranberry Chutney.................... 60

Brown Sugar Apple Dip........................... 60

Buffalo Chicken Dip 61

Buffalo Wings 62

Cereal Snack Mix with Salt-free
Seasoning 62

Chicken Nuggets with Honey Mustard
Dipping Sauce 63

Chicken Parmesan Meatballs 64

Chicken Pepper Bacon Wraps 64

Crispy-Crunch Snack Bars 65

Falafel 66

Flour Tortilla Chips 67

Garlic Oyster Crackers 67

Lemon Pepper Hummus 68

Pickled Okra 68

Raspberry Wings 69

SALADS & SALAD DRESSINGS..**69**

Apple Cranberry Slaw with Celery Seed
Dressing... 69

Asian Cabbage Slaw................................. 69

Basil-Lime Pineapple Fruit Salad 70

Broccoli and Apple Salad.......................... 71

Carrot and Jicama Salad 71

Celery Seed Dressing 72

Chicken Apple Crunch Salad 72

Cranberry Dijon Vinaigrette Dressing 73

Creamy Cucumber Salad........................... 73

Creamy Fruit Salad.................................... 74

Green Pepper Slaw 74

Grilled Chicken Salad 75

Lettuce and Mushroom Salad.................... 75

Lime Caribbean Dressing 76

Marinated Cucumber Salad 76

Matilde's Tuna Salad................................. 77

Mexican Coleslaw 77

Peach Basil Vinaigrette Dressing 78

Pear and Cranberry Salad with Honey-
Ginger Dressing... 79

Roasted Carrot and Cauliflower Salad 79

Roasted Vegetable Salad 80

Tuna Pasta Salad.. 80

Tuna Veggie Salad 81

Watermelon and Cucumber Salad 82

White Egg Salad... 82

SEAFOOD...**83**

Baked Trout with Lemon and Dill 83

Broiled Cod with Cucumber Sauce 83

Broiled Haddock with Cucumber Salsa 96

Cilantro-Lime Cod 96

Citrus Salmon... 97

Crab Cakes 97

Creamy Baked Fish 98

Easy Shrimp in Garlic Sauce 99

Fish Fry with Seasoned Rice...................... 99

Fish Tacos 100

Grilled Mexican Swordfish Fillets........... 101

Grilled Salmon 101

Salmon Steaks with Herb Dressing.......... 102

Sheet Pan Salmon and Green Beans......... 102

Shrimp and Asparagus Linguini............... 103

Sole with Tarragon Cream Sauce............. 104

South of the Border Shrimp Cocktail....... 104

Spicy Seafood Étouffée 105

Thai Pineapple Shrimp and Jasmine Rice 106

Tuna Ceviche... 106

Tuna Noodle Casserole for Two 107

CHICKEN AND TURKEY 108

Asian-Style Turkey Bowls 108

Cabbage Rolls Made with Turkey 108

Caribbean Curry Turkey 109

Chicken and Apple Curry......................... 110

Chicken and Rice Casserole..................... 110

Chicken in Rosemary-Garlic Sauce 111

Chicken in Wine Sauce 112

Chicken with Apples, Carrots, and
Grains 112

Chicken with Provencal Sauce................. 113

Chicken with Quinoa and Wild Rice 114

Easy Chicken and Pasta Dinner 114

Easy Chicken Breasts in Herb Sauce for
Two.. 115

Easy Chicken Enchiladas 116

Easy Crispy Lemon Chicken.................... 116

Garlic Chicken with Balsamic Vinegar.... 117

Glazed Cornish Game Hen for Two......... 117

Grilled Buttermilk Garlic Marinated
Chicken... 118

Grilled Chicken, Asparagus, and Corn..... 119

Homemade Chicken and Dumplings (or
Turkey) 119

Honey Mustard Grilled Chicken 120

BEEF AND LAMB..121

Asian Lettuce Wraps................................. 121

Beef Burgundy Crepes 121

Chinese Hotdish (Casserole).................... 121

Chipotle-Glazed Mini Meat Loaves......... 122

Cream Cheesy Burgers............................. 122

Easy BBQ Beef 123

Ground Beef and Green Pea Stove-top Casserole 124

Ground Beef and Veggie Foil Pack Dinner 124

SAUCES & SEASONINGS **127**

Adobo Seasoning................................ 127

Alfredo Sauce 127

Basic Meat Coating Mix 127

Basic White Sauce 127

Basil Pesto 128

Beef Brisket Gravy.............................. 128

Blackberry Sauce 129

Cucumber Dill Salsa............................ 129

Slow Roasted Beef Pot Roast with Carrots and Turnips 125

Southern Style Stuffed Peppers 125

Curried Onion and Garlic Seasoning........ 130

Garlic Sauce 130

Grilled Pineapple Salsa........................... 131

Blackberry Sauce 131

Cucumber Dill Salsa............................... 132

Curried Onion and Garlic Seasoning........ 132

Garlic Sauce 133

Grilled Pineapple Salsa........................... 133

SOUPS & STEWS **134**

Apple Cider Beef Stew........................ 134

Asian Soup Jar.................................... 134

Cabbage Borscht 135

Chicken Chili...................................... 136

Chicken Corn Soup................................ 136

Chicken Noodle Soup............................. 137

Chicken Wild Rice Soup 138

Moroccan Chicken Soup 138

BEVERAGES **140**

Almond Vanilla Espresso.......................... 140

Champagne Punch.................................... 140

Chocolate Smoothie 140

High Protein Piña Colada.......................... 140

High Protein Rice Milk 141

Homemade Rice Milk 141

Hot Apple Cider 142

Hot Holiday Cider (Low Sugar)............... 142

Lemon Cooler.. 143

Lemon Smoothie 143

Lemonade Cranberry Lime Protein Drink 144

30-DAY MEAL PLAN **144**

BONUS CHAPTER: INTERACTIVE TOOLS **147**

Daily Food and Fluid Intake Diary 147

Medication Management Worksheet 150

Blood Pressure Log 151

Lab Test Tracker 153

Symptom Tracker 155

Exercise Log 157

Appointment and Questions Tracker 158

Mood and Well-being Journal 161

Emergency Contact Sheet 163

CONCLUSION..**165**

INTRODUCTION

Janet's days flowed like a familiar melody through the streets of her New York neighborhood, a tune composed of early morning walks in Central Park, the laughter of her grandchildren echoing through her apartment, and the comforting aroma of her famous apple pie cooling on the windowsill. At 65, she had settled into a rhythm that felt as comforting as a well-worn quilt, each patch representing a cherished memory, a challenge overcome, a moment of joy shared with those she loved.

Her apartment, a cozy haven amidst the city's hustle, was filled with tokens of a life richly lived: photographs capturing moments of unguarded joy, souvenirs from family vacations, and, most importantly, the ever-present laughter and chatter of her family. Janet's role as the matriarch was undisputed; she was the glue that held them together, the storyteller of their collective history, the architect of their traditions.

But life, in its unpredictable wisdom, decided to add an unexpected chapter to Janet's story. A routine visit to the doctor, prompted by what she assumed were just signs of aging, revealed a truth that brought her world to a standstill: stage 4 kidney disease. The words felt foreign, an intruder in her carefully curated life, threatening to unravel the tapestry she had so lovingly woven.

The initial shock was palpable, a heavy silence that filled the room as Janet processed the news. But as the reality settled in, so did a familiar determination. Janet had faced challenges before—raising two children on her own, navigating the loss of loved ones, adapting to the ever-changing landscape of her beloved city. Each time, she emerged stronger, her spirit unbroken, her resolve unwavering.

This time was no different. Janet refused to let her diagnosis dictate the terms of her life. Instead, she approached it as she did everything else: with a blend of pragmatism and optimism. Her grandchildren, who had always seen their grandmother as invincible, now witnessed her vulnerability. Yet, in this vulnerability, they discovered a new depth of strength.

When Janet faced the stark reality of her diagnosis, she knew the path ahead required more than just determination; it needed expertise, especially in crafting a diet that could navigate the complexities of stage 4 kidney disease. It was then she remembered Hilda, a dietician and a close friend of her late daughter. Hilda, who had built a reputation in New York for her compassionate approach to nutritional therapy, was the first person Janet thought of in her quest for guidance.

Reaching out to Hilda wasn't easy. The weight of the news, coupled with the years that had passed since they last spoke, made Janet hesitant. However, the need for a familiar face, someone who understood the nuances of her life and loss, propelled her to make the call. Hilda, upon hearing from Janet after so many years, was initially taken aback. The news of Janet's condition struck a chord, reminding her of the fragility of life and the bonds that tie us to one another.

The reunion was a blend of emotions—joy at seeing each other after so long, and a shared sorrow for the reason behind it. Hilda, with her expertise and Janet's unwavering spirit, embarked on a journey to tailor a diet that not only met the strict requirements of kidney care but also brought joy and flavor back into Janet's life.

Together, they transformed Janet's kitchen into a place of healing and discovery. Hilda introduced Janet to the concept of "nutritional therapy," a way to manage her condition through food, which was both an art and a science. They spent hours discussing ingredients, swapping out sodium-heavy seasonings for herbs and spices that brought dishes to life without compromising Janet's health.

Hilda crafted interactive worksheets for Janet, a tool to track her dietary intake, symptoms, and overall well-being. These worksheets were more than just records; they were a tangible reflection of Janet's journey, filled with notes in the margins about new recipes they tried, adjustments to meals based on how she felt, and even little victories, like a return of her appetite or a particularly good day.

As the weeks turned into months, Janet began to notice a tangible shift in her health and well-being. The meticulous attention to her diet, guided by Hilda's expertise, had not only stabilized her condition but also imbued her with a newfound vitality. It was during one of their reflective afternoon sessions, amidst the clutter of recipe notes and worksheets on Janet's kitchen table, that an idea took root—an idea that would extend the warmth and wisdom of Janet's kitchen to others walking the same challenging path.

The decision to reach out to Hilda was made with a heavy heart and a deep sense of purpose. Janet knew that the book would be a tribute not only to their friendship and collaboration but also to the memory of her daughter, whose spirit had indirectly brought them together in this cause. With a mixture of apprehension and hope, Janet dialed Hilda's number, her fingers trembling slightly as she awaited the familiar voice on the other end.

The conversation that followed was a blend of tears, laughter, and long pauses filled with unspoken understanding. Hilda, moved by the proposal and touched by the thought of their shared efforts reaching a wider audience, gave her blessing without hesitation. The book, they decided, would be more than a compilation of kidney-friendly recipes; it would be a narrative of resilience, a guide infused with personal anecdotes, practical advice, and the emotional support needed to navigate the complexities of kidney disease in senior years.

Thus, the concept of "Stage 4 Kidney Disease Cookbook for Seniors" was born. It was a project rooted in the real-life experiences of two women united by circumstance and bound by a shared commitment to making a difference. The book was envisioned as a resource that would not only offer nutritional guidance but also serve as a companion to seniors and their families, providing comfort and encouragement through the stories of Janet and Hilda's journey.

In seeking Hilda's permission, Janet had bridged the final gap between the personal and the universal, turning their individual story into a collective source of hope. The book, once published, became a testament to the idea that even in our most challenging moments, we have the opportunity to contribute to something greater than ourselves, to offer a helping hand to those walking a similar path.

"Stage 4 Kidney Disease Cookbook for Seniors" thus stands as a beacon of hope, a reminder of the power of friendship, the importance of health, and the transformative potential of sharing one's journey. It is a moral tale that underscores the value of compassion, the impact of knowledge, and the enduring strength found in the bonds we forge, reminding us that together, we can face even the most daunting challenges.

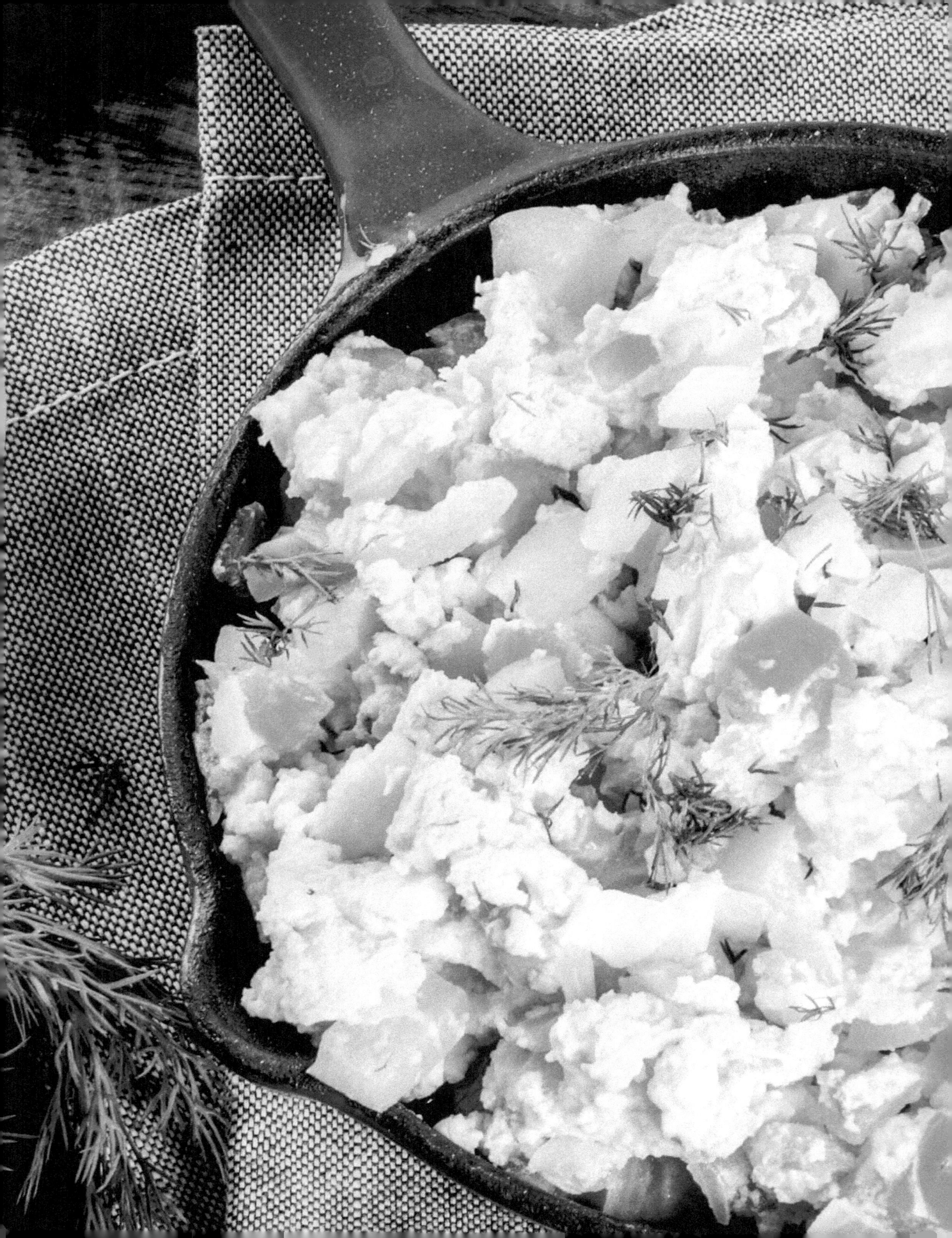

UNDERSTANDING STAGE 4 KIDNEY DISEASE

What Stage 4 Kidney Disease Really Means

Stage 4 kidney disease, a critical phase in the spectrum of chronic kidney disease (CKD), signifies a severe reduction in kidney function. This stage is characterized by a glomerular filtration rate (GFR) of 15-29 ml/min, indicating that the kidneys are operating at less than 30% of their normal function. At this juncture, the kidneys can no longer efficiently perform their vital roles—filtering waste from the blood, regulating blood pressure, balancing electrolytes, and producing red blood cells.

The implications of Stage 4 kidney disease are profound. It's a harbinger of end-stage renal disease (ESRD), where kidney function is so diminished that dialysis or a kidney transplant becomes necessary to sustain life. However, reaching Stage 4 does not mean the battle is lost. With appropriate management, the progression to ESRD can be delayed, offering patients valuable time and quality of life.

Understanding this stage is crucial for patients and caregivers alike. It demands a proactive approach to health management, including stringent control of blood pressure, careful management of diabetes, dietary modifications, and regular consultations with healthcare providers. It's a stage that calls for resilience, adaptation, and an informed partnership between patients and their medical teams.

Root Causes and Contributing Factors to Stage 4

The journey to Stage 4 kidney disease is often paved with a combination of genetic, environmental, and lifestyle factors. Understanding these can offer insights into prevention and management strategies.

1. **Diabetes**: The leading cause of CKD, diabetes, particularly type 2, wreaks havoc on the kidneys through high blood sugar levels. Over time, this can damage the vessels in the kidneys, impairing their ability to filter waste.

2. **High Blood Pressure**: Another major contributor, high blood pressure, can cause damage to the blood vessels in the kidneys, reducing their filtering capabilities. Managing blood pressure is paramount in slowing the progression of CKD.

3. **Glomerulonephritis**: This group of diseases involves the inflammation of the glomeruli, the filtering units of the kidneys. It can be acute or chronic and is a common pathway to CKD.

4. **Polycystic Kidney Disease**: A genetic disorder characterized by the growth of numerous cysts in the kidneys, compromising their function over time.

5. **Prolonged Obstruction of the Urinary Tract**: Conditions such as enlarged prostate, kidney stones, and some cancers can lead to blockages that, if not treated, can cause significant kidney damage.

6. **Recurrent Kidney Infection**: Repeated infections can lead to scarring and loss of kidney function.

7. **Lifestyle Factors**: Smoking, obesity, and excessive use of NSAIDs can contribute to the risk of developing CKD.

Each of these factors can independently or in combination with others, led to the deterioration of kidney function, culminating in Stage 4 CKD. Early detection and management of these risk factors are critical in preventing or slowing the progression of kidney disease.

Symptoms of Stage 4

The symptoms of Stage 4 kidney disease are often more pronounced than in the earlier stages, reflecting the significant loss of kidney function. Recognizing these symptoms is crucial for timely intervention.

1. **Fatigue and Weakness**: As waste accumulates in the blood, patients may experience persistent fatigue and a general feeling of weakness, often due to anemia associated with reduced erythropoietin production by the kidneys.

2. **Changes in Urination**: This can include increased frequency, especially at night, difficulty urinating, or foamy or dark urine, indicating the kidneys' struggle to filter and balance fluids.

3. **Swelling (Edema)**: Reduced kidney function can lead to fluid retention, causing swelling in the legs, ankles, feet, face, or hands.

4. **Nausea and Vomiting**: The buildup of toxins in the blood can lead to gastrointestinal symptoms, including a loss of appetite, nausea, and vomiting.

5. **High Blood Pressure**: Difficulty in managing blood pressure can be both a cause and a symptom of progressing kidney disease.

6. **Cognitive Impairments**: Toxins affecting the brain can lead to difficulties with concentration, dizziness, and, in severe cases, seizures.

7. **Shortness of Breath**: Fluid buildup in the lungs, a result of the kidneys' reduced ability to manage fluid balance, can cause breathing difficulties.

8.

NUTRITIONAL GUIDELINES FOR STAGE 4 CKD IN SENIORS

The Foundation of Disease Management in Stage 4 Kidney Disease

Managing Stage 4 Chronic Kidney Disease (CKD) is akin to navigating a complex network of highways, each path requiring careful consideration, preparation, and sometimes, the courage to take the road less traveled. At this advanced stage, where the kidneys operate at significantly reduced efficiency, the foundation of disease management is built on a multidisciplinary approach that addresses the multifaceted challenges patients face. This comprehensive strategy not only aims to slow the progression of the disease but also to enhance the quality of life for those living with Stage 4 CKD.

Personalized Care Plans: Tailoring Treatment to the Individual

The cornerstone of effective disease management in Stage 4 CKD is the development of a personalized care plan. This tailored approach takes into account the unique medical history, lifestyle, and personal preferences of each patient, ensuring that the treatment strategy is as individualized as the patients themselves. Key components of this personalized care plan include:

1. **Medical Management**: Central to slowing the progression of CKD is the meticulous management of underlying conditions such as diabetes and hypertension, which are often the culprits behind kidney damage. This involves a regimented approach to medication adherence, regular monitoring of blood sugar and blood pressure levels, and adjustments to treatment protocols as necessary.

2. **Dietary Modifications**: Nutrition plays a pivotal role in managing Stage 4 CKD. Patients are often advised to adopt a kidney-friendly diet that limits the intake of sodium, potassium, and phosphorus, nutrients that overburdened kidneys struggle to filter effectively. A registered dietitian specializing in renal diets can provide invaluable guidance, helping patients navigate the complexities of nutritional management while ensuring their meals remain enjoyable and satisfying.

3. **Fluid Intake Regulation**: As the kidneys' ability to balance fluid levels diminishes, careful monitoring of fluid intake becomes crucial. Patients are often counseled to adhere to a fluid restriction to prevent the complications associated with fluid overload, including hypertension, swelling, and heart failure.

4. **Lifestyle Adjustments**: Engaging in regular, moderate exercise, quitting smoking, and maintaining a healthy weight are all integral parts of managing Stage 4 CKD. These lifestyle adjustments not only support overall health but can also mitigate the risk factors contributing to kidney disease progression.

Multidisciplinary Support: A Team Approach to Comprehensive Care

Effective management of Stage 4 CKD requires the collaboration of a multidisciplinary team dedicated to providing comprehensive care. This team typically includes nephrologists, dietitians, nurses, pharmacists, and social workers, each playing a distinct role in supporting the patient's journey through CKD management.

1. **Nephrologists**: Specialists in kidney care, nephrologists oversee the medical management of CKD, coordinating care and guiding patients through treatment options, including the potential need for dialysis or kidney transplantation.
2. **Dietitians**: Expertise in renal nutrition is crucial for managing the dietary challenges of CKD. Dietitians work closely with patients to develop meal plans that meet their nutritional needs while adhering to dietary restrictions.
3. **Nurses and Pharmacists**: Nurses provide ongoing education, support, and care coordination, while pharmacists assist with medication management, ensuring that patients understand their regimens and potential side effects.
4. **Social Workers**: The emotional and psychological impact of living with Stage 4 CKD cannot be understated. Social workers offer counseling and support, helping patients navigate the complexities of chronic illness, including financial and social challenges.

Role of Proteins in Kidney Disease Management

Proteins, the building blocks of life, are essential for the growth, repair, and maintenance of all body tissues. They play critical roles in the formation of enzymes, hormones, and other vital substances. However, the metabolism of proteins generates nitrogenous waste products, primarily urea, which the kidneys filter out from the blood and excrete in the urine. In healthy individuals, this process is efficiently managed, but in those with CKD, the kidneys' ability to excrete these waste products is compromised, leading to their accumulation in the blood—a condition known as uremia.

The management of protein intake in CKD patients is a balancing act. On one hand, adequate protein is necessary to prevent malnutrition, preserve muscle mass, and maintain overall health. On the other hand, excessive protein intake can exacerbate kidney damage by increasing the burden on already compromised kidneys. The key lies in optimizing the amount and type of protein consumed, a strategy that requires careful planning and monitoring.

Low-Protein Diets

Research has shown that a low-protein diet can help slow the progression of CKD and delay the onset of end-stage renal disease (ESRD). By reducing the intake of protein, the production of urea and other nitrogenous wastes is decreased, thereby lessening the kidneys' workload and the accumulation of toxins in the blood. This dietary approach can also help manage symptoms such as fatigue, nausea, and poor appetite, contributing to an improved quality of life.

However, the implementation of a low-protein diet must be carefully managed to avoid the risk of malnutrition. Patients are often advised to consume high-quality proteins—those containing all the essential amino acids—in moderate amounts. Sources of high-quality protein include lean meats, fish, eggs, and dairy products. Plant-based proteins, while beneficial for overall health, may need to be supplemented with other protein sources to ensure a complete amino acid profile.

The Emerging Perspective on Plant-Based Diets

Recent studies suggest that plant-based diets may offer additional benefits for CKD patients beyond protein management. These diets are typically lower in protein compared to diets that include meat and are rich in anti-inflammatory compounds and antioxidants, which can help reduce stress on the kidneys. Furthermore, plant-based diets are associated with lower blood pressure and improved blood sugar control, factors that are crucial in managing CKD.

Given the individual variability in CKD progression, dietary protein needs can differ significantly from one patient to another. Factors such as the stage of kidney disease, the presence of other health conditions, and the patient's nutritional status must all be considered when devising a dietary plan. This underscores the importance of working with a renal dietitian, a specialist who can tailor dietary recommendations to meet the specific needs of each patient, ensuring adequate nutrition while minimizing the risk to kidney health.

Micromanagement of Micronutrients in Kidney Disease

Micronutrients include vitamins and minerals, essential elements that support a myriad of physiological functions—from bone health and immune function to blood clotting and energy production. In CKD, the kidneys' ability to regulate these nutrients is compromised, leading to deficiencies or toxicities that can significantly affect a patient's health and quality of life.

Vitamins in CKD

Vitamins are organic compounds that the body needs in small amounts for various metabolic processes. In CKD, the management of certain vitamins becomes crucial:

1. **Vitamin D**: The kidneys convert vitamin D into its active form, which is vital for calcium absorption and bone health. CKD often leads to vitamin D deficiency, necessitating careful supplementation to prevent bone disorders and maintain calcium-phosphate balance.
2. **Vitamin C**: While essential for immune function and as an antioxidant, excessive vitamin C can lead to oxalate accumulation in CKD patients, increasing the risk of kidney stones. Thus, a balance must be struck to avoid deficiency without risking toxicity.
3. **B Vitamins**: Particularly B6, B12, and folic acid, play roles in red blood cell formation and the prevention of anemia, a common complication in CKD. Supplementation can help manage anemia but requires monitoring to avoid adverse effects.

Minerals in CKD

Minerals are inorganic elements that also play critical roles in bodily functions. Their management in CKD is complex due to the kidneys' impaired ability to excrete or retain these elements as needed:

1. **Potassium**: Essential for nerve function and muscle contraction, including the heart. CKD can lead to hyperkalemia (high potassium levels), which poses risks of cardiac issues. Dietary potassium must be carefully managed to avoid these risks.
2. **Phosphorus**: While vital for energy production and bone health, CKD often leads to hyperphosphatemia (high phosphorus levels), contributing to bone disease and vascular calcification. Phosphorus intake must be limited, and binders may be used to control its levels in the blood.
3. **Calcium**: The balance of calcium is intricately linked with phosphorus and vitamin D. In CKD, calcium supplementation must be carefully managed to prevent vascular calcification while supporting bone health.

4. **Iron**: Iron deficiency is common in CKD due to reduced erythropoietin production and the loss of blood during hemodialysis. Iron supplementation can help manage anemia but requires monitoring to prevent iron overload.

Micronutrient Management Strategies

The management of micronutrients in CKD involves a delicate balance, tailored to the individual's disease stage, dietary restrictions, and overall health profile. Strategies include:

- **Dietary Adjustments**: A dietitian specializing in CKD can provide guidance on food choices that meet nutritional needs without exacerbating kidney damage. This may involve limiting certain foods high in phosphorus, potassium, or sodium while ensuring adequate intake of other essential nutrients.
- **Supplementation**: In cases where dietary adjustments cannot fully address micronutrient imbalances, supplements may be prescribed. These must be carefully selected and dosed to avoid toxicity, particularly for fat-soluble vitamins and minerals that the body cannot easily excrete.
- **Regular Monitoring**: Blood tests are essential to monitor levels of key micronutrients, allowing for adjustments in diet or supplementation as needed. This ongoing monitoring is crucial to prevent complications associated with both deficiencies and excesses.
- **Education and Empowerment**: Patients and caregivers must be educated about the importance of micronutrient management in CKD. Understanding the role of diet, the potential need for supplements, and the signs of micronutrient imbalances can empower patients to take an active role in their care.

Role Fluids in Kidney Disease

In the context of kidney disease, fluids can be seen as a double-edged sword. On one hand, adequate hydration is crucial for the kidneys to perform their primary function—filtering waste from the blood and excreting it in the urine. On the other hand, when kidney function is impaired, particularly in the advanced stages of kidney disease, the kidneys' ability to manage fluid balance is compromised. This can lead to fluid overload, a condition where the body retains more fluid than it excretes, resulting in swelling (edema), high blood pressure, and added strain on the heart.

Navigating Fluid Intake in Kidney Disease

The management of fluid intake is a critical aspect of living with kidney disease. It requires a nuanced understanding of the body's needs, the stage of kidney disease, and the individual's overall health profile. Here's how fluid management plays out across different stages of kidney disease:

1. **Early Stages of Kidney Disease**: In the initial stages, the kidneys often retain much of their ability to manage fluids. Patients may not need to drastically alter their fluid intake but should be mindful of consuming excessive amounts of fluids, especially those high in sugars, sodium, and other additives that can exacerbate kidney damage.

2. **Advanced Kidney Disease and Dialysis**: As kidney disease progresses to Stage 4 and beyond, the situation changes significantly. Patients may need to limit their fluid intake to prevent fluid overload. For those on dialysis, especially hemodialysis, fluid restrictions become a critical part of their daily regimen. Dialysis can only remove a certain amount of fluid at each session, making it essential to avoid drinking more fluid than the body can handle between treatments.

The Impact of Fluid Type

Not all fluids are created equal, especially when it comes to kidney health. Here are some considerations for choosing the right types of fluids:

- **Water**: The best choice for hydration, water is free of calories, sugars, and additives. It helps to flush out toxins and supports overall kidney function.
- **High-Sodium Fluids**: Soups, broths, and beverages high in sodium can increase blood pressure and fluid retention, posing risks for kidney patients.
- **Sugary Drinks**: Sodas, fruit juices, and other sugary drinks can contribute to obesity and diabetes, two major risk factors for kidney disease.
- **Alcohol and Caffeine**: Both can have diuretic effects, leading to dehydration. In moderation, they may be acceptable for some patients, but it's essential to consult with a healthcare provider.

Monitoring and Managing Fluid Intake

Effective fluid management in kidney disease involves careful monitoring and adjustments based on several factors, including urine output, thirst, and the presence of edema. Here are some strategies for managing fluid intake:

- **Measure Your Intake**: Keeping a daily log of fluid intake can help patients stay within their recommended limits.
- **Understand Your Fluid Needs**: These can vary based on activity level, climate, and health status. Regular consultations with a healthcare provider can help determine the right balance.
- **Manage Thirst**: Sipping water throughout the day, sucking on ice chips, or using sugar-free gum can help manage thirst without exceeding fluid intake limits.
- **Be Mindful of Hidden Fluids**: Foods like soups, ice cream, and fruits also contribute to total fluid intake and should be considered in daily calculations.

Role of Fiber and Antioxidants in Kidney Disease

Dietary fiber, a complex carbohydrate found in plant foods, is known for its benefits to digestive health. However, its advantages extend far beyond aiding digestion, especially for individuals with kidney disease. Fiber's role in kidney health can be understood through several key mechanisms:

1. **Regulation of Blood Sugar Levels**: For those with diabetes, a leading cause of kidney disease, fiber helps slow down glucose absorption, aiding in blood sugar control. This regulation is crucial in minimizing the risk of further kidney damage.

2. **Reduction of Blood Pressure**: High blood pressure is another major risk factor for kidney disease. A diet high in fiber has been associated with lower blood pressure levels, likely due to fiber's ability to improve arterial function and reduce systemic inflammation.

3. **Cholesterol Management**: Fiber helps lower LDL (bad) cholesterol levels, reducing the risk of atherosclerosis (hardening of the arteries), which can compromise kidney health by affecting the renal arteries.

4. **Gut Health and Uremic Toxins**: Fiber plays a vital role in maintaining gut health. It promotes the growth of beneficial gut bacteria, which can help reduce the production and absorption of uremic toxins—harmful substances that can accumulate in the blood as kidney function declines.

Incorporating fiber into the diet of someone with kidney disease requires a careful balance. While beneficial, too much fiber can lead to gastrointestinal discomfort and, in cases where potassium and phosphorus intake needs to be monitored, not all high-fiber foods may be suitable. Sources like berries, carrots, and chia seeds can provide fiber without excessively increasing potassium and phosphorus levels.

Antioxidants: The Protective Shield

Antioxidants are compounds that help neutralize free radicals—unstable molecules that can cause cellular damage, contributing to chronic diseases, including kidney disease. The protective role of antioxidants is particularly relevant for individuals with kidney disease, as oxidative stress is both a contributor to and a consequence of kidney damage.

1. **Combating Oxidative Stress**: Antioxidants like vitamins C and E, selenium, and flavonoids can help reduce oxidative stress by neutralizing free radicals. This reduction is crucial in slowing the progression of kidney disease.

2. **Inflammation Reduction**: Chronic inflammation is a hallmark of kidney disease. Antioxidants have anti-inflammatory properties that can help mitigate this inflammation, protecting kidney cells from further damage.

3. **Enhancing Immune Function**: Kidney disease can compromise the immune system, making individuals more susceptible to infections. Antioxidants can strengthen the immune response, offering additional protection.

4. **Supporting Overall Kidney Function**: By reducing oxidative stress and inflammation, antioxidants can help preserve kidney function, potentially delaying the progression to end-stage renal disease.

Sources of antioxidants suitable for those with kidney disease include bell peppers, apples, and blueberries, which provide a high antioxidant content without significantly impacting potassium and phosphorus levels.

Incorporating Fiber and Antioxidants into a Kidney-Friendly Diet

Adopting a diet rich in fiber and antioxidants requires thoughtful planning, especially for those with advanced kidney disease. Here are some strategies:

- **Choose Low-Potassium Fruits and Vegetables**: Opt for fruits and vegetables that are lower in potassium if this is a concern. Apples, berries, and bell peppers are excellent choices.

- **Incorporate Whole Grains**: Select whole grains that are lower in phosphorus, such as bulgur, buckwheat, and wild rice, to increase fiber intake.

- **Use Herbs and Spices**: Enhance the flavor of dishes with herbs and spices, many of which are rich in antioxidants, instead of relying on salt.

- **Monitor Portion Sizes**: Keep an eye on portion sizes to manage the intake of nutrients like potassium and phosphorus effectively.

MEAL PLANNING AND PREPARATION

Creating a Kidney-Friendly Kitchen

Stocking Up on Kidney-Friendly Staples

The foundation of a kidney-friendly kitchen lies in its pantry and refrigerator contents. Prioritizing low-sodium, low-potassium, and low-phosphorus foods while ensuring a balanced intake of proteins and other nutrients is key. Here's how to stock up smartly:

- **Grains and Cereals**: Opt for whole grains like barley, buckwheat, and bulgur. These provide essential B vitamins and fiber without overloading your system with phosphorus found in processed grains.
- **Fruits and Vegetables**: Fresh is best, but when that's not possible, look for frozen options without added sauces or seasonings. Apples, berries, carrots, and green beans are excellent choices. Remember, some fruits and vegetables are high in potassium and should be limited or avoided.
- **Protein Sources**: High-quality proteins are crucial. Fresh cuts of beef, chicken, and pork, as well as egg whites, provide protein without excessive phosphorus. For plant-based proteins, consider lentils and chickpeas, but be mindful of portion sizes to manage potassium levels.
- **Dairy Alternatives**: Since dairy products can be high in phosphorus, explore alternatives like almond milk or rice milk, ensuring they are unenriched with phosphates.
- **Herbs and Spices**: To reduce sodium intake, stock up on a variety of herbs and spices. Fresh or dried, they can transform any dish without the need for salt.

Tools and Equipment for Easy and Safe Meal Preparation

Equipping your kitchen with the right tools can make meal preparation easier, safer, and more enjoyable. Consider these essentials:

- **High-Quality Knives**: A set of sharp knives makes chopping and slicing less laborious, especially for those with arthritis or limited hand strength.
- **Slow Cooker**: Ideal for tenderizing tougher cuts of meat while infusing flavors without added salt or fat.
- **Steamer Basket**: Steaming preserves nutrients in vegetables better than boiling and requires no added fats.
- **Spice Grinder or Mortar and Pestle**: Freshly grinding herbs and spices maximizes flavor, allowing you to create your own salt-free seasoning blends.

- **Measuring Cups and Spoons**: Essential for controlling portion sizes and ensuring accurate nutrient intake.

Organizing Your Kitchen for Efficiency and Accessibility

A well-organized kitchen saves time, reduces stress, and makes cooking a more enjoyable experience. Here are some tips to keep your kitchen orderly and accessible:

- **Label Everything**: Use clear labels on containers and shelves to make it easy to find what you need. Consider using large print or color-coding for those with visual impairments.
- **Keep Frequently Used Items Within Reach**: Store everyday items on lower shelves and in front drawers to minimize bending and stretching.
- **Declutter the Counters**: Keep only essential items on countertops to create a spacious, functional workspace.
- **Use Drawer Organizers**: These can help keep utensils and small tools neatly arranged and easy to find.

Creating a Safe Cooking Environment

Safety in the kitchen is paramount, especially for seniors. Implement these measures to prevent accidents and injuries:

- **Ensure Good Lighting**: Adequate lighting reduces the risk of cuts and falls. Consider adding under-cabinet lights for better visibility.
- **Install Non-Slip Mats**: Place these in front of the sink, stove, and prep areas to help prevent slips and falls.
- **Use Automatic Shut-Off Appliances**: Look for kitchen appliances with safety features like automatic shut-offs to avoid accidents.
- **Keep a Fire Extinguisher Handy**: Make sure it's easily accessible and that you know how to use it.

Embracing Technology for Meal Planning and Nutrition Tracking

Technology can be a valuable ally in managing your kidney-friendly diet. Numerous apps and online resources are available to help plan meals, track nutrient intake, and even deliver groceries to your doorstep. Explore apps that specialize in dietary management for kidney disease, offering features like personalized meal planning, grocery lists, and nutritional analysis.

Designing Your Meal Plan

At the heart of managing Stage 4 Kidney Disease is understanding the delicate balance of nutrients essential for maintaining optimal health. This balance involves limiting certain nutrients such as sodium, potassium, phosphorus, and protein, which, when kidneys are compromised, can accumulate in the body and cause harm. However, the goal is not just to limit but to nourish, ensuring that each meal is a building block towards better health.

Step 1: Understanding Nutritional Guidelines

The first step in designing your meal plan is to familiarize yourself with the nutritional guidelines specific to Stage 4 Kidney Disease. Collaborating with a healthcare provider or dietitian can provide personalized advice based on your health status, dietary needs, and preferences. This personalized approach ensures that the meal plan supports your kidney health without compromising on taste or variety.

Step 2: Incorporating Variety and Balance

A common misconception about kidney-friendly diets is that they are restrictive and monotonous. However, with a bit of creativity and planning, you can enjoy a diverse and flavorful diet. Start by listing kidney-friendly foods that you enjoy and those you're curious to try. This list will serve as the foundation for your meal plan, ensuring that you have a variety of options to keep meals interesting and enjoyable.

Fruits and Vegetables: Opt for low-potassium choices like apples, berries, carrots, and green beans. These can be incorporated into meals and snacks throughout the day.

Grains: Choose whole grains that are lower in phosphorus, such as bulgur wheat, buckwheat, and rice. These grains can serve as the base for many dishes, from salads to stir-fries.

Proteins: Focus on high-quality, low-phosphorus protein sources like egg whites, poultry, and fish. Remember, portion control is key to managing protein intake.

Dairy: Opt for alternatives like almond milk or rice milk, which are lower in phosphorus and potassium than traditional dairy products.

Step 3: Planning for the Week

With a list of kidney-friendly foods in hand, the next step is to start planning your meals for the week. This involves deciding what you'll eat for each meal and snack, ensuring that you have a balanced intake of nutrients throughout the day. A weekly meal plan helps in managing your grocery shopping more efficiently, reducing waste, and alleviating the daily stress of deciding what to eat.

Breakfast Ideas: Start your day with a nourishing meal, such as a bowl of low-phosphorus cereal with almond milk, topped with fresh berries.

Lunch Ideas: Prepare a hearty salad with mixed greens, shredded chicken, and a variety of vegetables. Dress it with a homemade vinaigrette made with olive oil and lemon juice.

Dinner Ideas: Enjoy a piece of grilled fish with a side of roasted carrots and a serving of bulgur wheat for a balanced and satisfying meal.

Snack Ideas: Keep snacks simple and kidney-friendly, like apple slices with almond butter or a small serving of homemade trail mix with dried cranberries and almonds.

Step 4: Adapting Recipes and Meals

Adapting your favorite recipes to fit a kidney-friendly diet can make meal planning more enjoyable. This might involve substituting certain ingredients or adjusting cooking methods to reduce sodium, potassium, and phosphorus content. For example, using herbs and spices instead of salt to flavor dishes, or choosing fresh or frozen produce over canned to avoid added sodium and preservatives.

Step 5: Meal Prepping and Batch Cooking

Meal prepping and batch cooking are invaluable strategies for managing a kidney-friendly diet, especially for seniors. Preparing meals in advance can save time, reduce stress, and ensure that you have healthy options readily available. Dedicate a day to cooking and portioning out meals for the week, storing them in the refrigerator or freezer for easy reheating.

Smart Shopping Strategies

Understanding Food Labels: The First Line of Defense

The journey to smart shopping begins with mastering the art of reading food labels. These labels are your first line of defense against hidden dietary dangers, offering crucial insights into the nutritional content of foods. For those with kidney disease, the focus should be on key nutrients: sodium, potassium, phosphorus, and protein.

- **Sodium**: Look for low-sodium or no-salt-added options. Remember, 'reduced sodium' does not mean low sodium; it simply contains less sodium than the original product.
- **Potassium**: While potassium content isn't always listed, be cautious with potassium-rich foods like bananas, oranges, and potatoes. Opt for fresh or frozen fruits and vegetables, as canned versions often have added potassium for preservation.
- **Phosphorus**: Phosphorus is rarely listed on food labels, making it tricky to track. As a general rule, avoid processed foods and sodas, as they often contain added phosphorus.
- **Protein**: While essential, protein intake needs to be moderated in Stage 4 Kidney Disease. Choose lean protein sources and be mindful of portion sizes.

The Art of the Shopping List

A well-thought-out shopping list is your blueprint for navigating the grocery store. Start by planning your meals for the week, considering the balance of nutrients necessary for your diet. Your list should categorize items by section (produce, dairy, meats, etc.) to streamline your shopping experience and reduce the temptation of impulse buys.

Incorporate a variety of fruits, vegetables, whole grains, and lean proteins into your list, ensuring you have a rainbow of nutrients to choose from. Remember, variety not only adds excitement to your meals but also helps cover the nutritional spectrum needed for a kidney-friendly diet.

Navigating Grocery Store Aisles

With list in hand, it's time to tackle the grocery store. Here are strategies to make your shopping trip efficient and effective:

- **Stick to the Perimeter**: Fresh produce, meats, and dairy are typically located around the store's edges. These areas are your go-to for the bulk of your shopping, offering the freshest and least processed options.
- **Venture Inward with Caution**: The inner aisles house canned goods, cereals, and other packaged foods. Here, vigilance is key. Opt for whole grain options, low-sodium broths, and canned vegetables with no added salt.
- **Read Labels Religiously**: Even with a shopping list, unexpected choices can arise. Use your knowledge of food labels to make informed decisions, keeping your dietary restrictions in mind.
- **Seek Out Special Sections**: Many stores have health-focused or international sections offering unique ingredients that fit within a kidney-friendly diet. These can be great sources for adding variety to your meals.

Cooking Techniques and Tips

1. **Steaming and Poaching**: These gentle cooking methods preserve the natural flavors of foods without the need for added fats or salts. Steaming vegetables, fish, and poultry can retain nutrients that might be lost in boiling. Poaching in a flavorful liquid, like a homemade low-sodium broth, can infuse dishes with depth and complexity.
2. **Sautéing with Broth**: Instead of using oil or butter, try sautéing with a small amount of vegetable broth or water. This method allows for the caramelization of ingredients like onions and garlic, which form the flavor foundation for countless dishes, without adding unnecessary fats or sodium.

3. **Roasting to Enhance Flavors**: Roasting can intensify the natural sweetness and flavors of vegetables and meats. To minimize the need for added salt, season your dishes with a mix of herbs and spices. Experiment with combinations like rosemary and garlic for potatoes or cumin and lime zest for carrots to discover new favorites.

4. **Utilizing Herbs and Spices**: The key to making kidney-friendly dishes burst with flavor lies in the liberal use of herbs and spices. Fresh herbs like basil, cilantro, and parsley can add a fresh pop to any dish, while dried spices can bring warmth and depth. Create your own salt-free seasoning blends to have on hand for easy flavoring.

5. **Acid Adds Zest**: A splash of acid, from vinegar or citrus juice, can brighten up any dish and reduce the need for salt. Lemon juice over sautéed greens, a dash of balsamic vinegar in soups, or a squeeze of lime in grain dishes can make flavors pop.

Adapting Recipes to Meet Dietary Needs

1. **Ingredient Swaps**: Get creative with substitutions that lower potassium, phosphorus, and sodium levels. Use white rice instead of brown to reduce phosphorus and potassium. Swap nuts and seeds in recipes with less phosphorus-dense options like unsalted popcorn or homemade low-sodium bread crumbs.

2. **Phosphorus and Potassium Management**: Cooking methods can impact the levels of certain minerals in your food. For example, double boiling potatoes and other root vegetables can help reduce their potassium content. Be mindful of ingredients like dairy, nuts, and whole grains, which are high in phosphorus, and seek alternatives or adjust portion sizes accordingly.

3. **Reducing Sodium**: Instead of salt, harness the power of flavor-packed ingredients like garlic, onion, and your arsenal of herbs and spices. Be wary of hidden sodium in canned goods and broths; opt for fresh or frozen vegetables and make your own stocks whenever possible.

Safe Food Handling and Preparation

1. **Cross-Contamination Awareness**: Keep raw and cooked foods separate, and use different cutting boards and utensils for meats and vegetables. This practice is crucial in preventing foodborne illnesses, which can be particularly harmful to individuals with compromised kidney function.

2. **Proper Storage**: Refrigerate perishable foods within two hours of cooking. Store leftovers in clear, airtight containers to keep them fresh and prevent any confusion about their contents or how long they've been stored.

3. **Mindful Tasting**: For those on a restricted diet, even tasting while cooking can add up in terms of sodium and potassium intake. Use small spoons and limit tasting to necessary checks for seasoning adjustments.

Eating Well Outside the Home

Dining out is one of life's pleasures, offering opportunities for socialization, celebration, and a break from the routine of home-cooked meals. However, for seniors managing Stage 4 Kidney Disease, the array of menu options can seem like a minefield, with hidden dangers of excessive sodium, potassium, and phosphorus lurking in seemingly innocuous dishes. The key to successfully navigating this landscape is preparation, knowledge, and communication.

Understanding Menu Descriptions

The first step in dining out safely is learning to decode menu descriptions. Words like "brined," "marinated," or "preserved" can indicate high sodium content, while "creamy," "cheesy," or "buttery" may signal dishes rich in phosphorus and potassium. Opting for "grilled," "baked," or "steamed" dishes can lead to healthier choices, as these cooking methods typically use less salt and fat. However, it's important to inquire about seasonings and cooking methods, as appearances can be deceiving.

Communicating Dietary Needs

Effective communication with restaurant staff is crucial. Don't hesitate to ask questions about menu items or request modifications to dishes. Most establishments are willing to accommodate dietary restrictions, such as preparing a dish without added salt or serving sauces and dressings on the side. Be specific about your needs, and consider calling ahead to discuss your dietary requirements with the chef or manager, especially if you plan to visit during peak hours when restaurants are busiest.

Choosing the Right Establishments

Some types of restaurants are more likely to offer kidney-friendly options than others. For example, establishments that emphasize fresh, whole foods and offer a variety of vegetable-based dishes are often a good choice. Ethnic restaurants, while offering a rich tapestry of flavors, can be challenging due to the liberal use of sauces and seasonings high in sodium, potassium, and phosphorus. Researching restaurants in advance and reading menus online can help you select the best options before you even leave home.

Portion Control and Sharing

Restaurant portions are frequently larger than what one might serve at home, making it easy to overindulge in foods that should be consumed in moderation. Consider sharing entrees with dining companions or asking for a half portion. Not only does this strategy help manage portion sizes, but it also allows you to enjoy a wider variety of dishes without exceeding dietary restrictions.

Beverage Choices

Beverages can also pose a challenge, as many drinks contain added sugars, sodium, and other additives that are best avoided. Opt for water, sparkling water, or unsweetened tea to stay hydrated without impacting your dietary goals. If you enjoy alcohol, discuss with your healthcare provider whether it's safe to include in your diet and, if so, what types and amounts are acceptable.

Navigating Social Gatherings

Social gatherings, from family celebrations to community events, can present similar challenges to dining out. When attending a potluck or dinner party, consider bringing a dish that meets your dietary needs. This not only ensures you'll have something safe to eat, but it also introduces others to the delicious possibilities of kidney-friendly cuisine.

When you're not in control of the menu, focus on the aspects of the meal you can manage, such as portion sizes and food choices. Fill your plate with the safest options available, such as lean proteins and non-starchy vegetables, and steer clear of dishes that are likely to be high in sodium, potassium, and phosphorus.

BREAKFAST

Apple Puffs

Prep Time: 1 hour Cooking Time: 20 minutes

Serving Size: 1 square

Ingredients:

- 1 can apple pie filling (21 oz)
- 1 tsp ground cinnamon
- ½ tsp rum extract
- 1⅓ sheets of puff pastry dough (8 oz)
- 1 tsp baking soda
- 1 tsp powdered sugar

Instructions:

1. Thaw puff pastry dough for 50-60 minutes at room temperature if frozen.
2. Preheat the oven to 400°F.
3. In a bowl, mix the apple pie filling with cinnamon and rum extract. If the apples are sliced, cut them into thirds.
4. Unfold one sheet of dough and cut into 9 equal squares. Use one-third of the dough from the other sheet and cut this section into 3 more equal squares.
5. Place each square into a muffin tin slot and spoon the apple filling into each.
6. Bake for 15 minutes or until golden brown.
7. Remove from muffin tins while warm and sprinkle powdered sugar on top before serving.

Nutritional Information (per serving):

- Calories: 156.5
- Protein: 1.5g
- Sodium: 176.5mg
- Potassium: 35mg
- Total Fat: 7.3g
- Saturated Fat: 1.7g
- Cholesterol: 0mg
- Carbohydrates: 22.5g
- Fiber: 1g

Banana Oat Shake

Prep Time: 5 minutes Cooking Time: Not applicable Serving Size: 1 serving

Ingredients:

- ¼ cup cooked oatmeal, chilled
- ⅓ cup skim milk
- 1 tbsp brown sugar
- ½ tbsp wheat germ
- ¾ tsp vanilla extract
- ¼ frozen banana, cut into chunks

Instructions:

1. Place the chilled oatmeal in a blender and blend for a few minutes to break it down.
2. Add the skim milk, brown sugar, wheat germ, vanilla extract, and frozen banana chunks to the blender.
3. Blend until the mixture is thick and smooth. Serve immediately, adding ice if desired for extra chill.

Nutritional Information (per serving):

- Calories: 172

- Protein: 6g
- Sodium: 42.5mg
- Potassium: 297.5mg
- Carbohydrates: 33g

Banana-Apple Smoothie

Prep Time: 5 minutes Cooking Time: Not applicable Serving Size: 1 serving

Ingredients:

- ½ banana, peeled & cut into chunks
- ½ cup plain yogurt
- ½ cup unsweetened applesauce
- ¼ cup skim milk
- 1 tbsp honey
- 2 tbsp oat bran

Instructions:

1. Place the banana, yogurt, applesauce, milk, and honey in a blender.
2. Blend until smooth.
3. Add the oat bran and blend again until the mixture is thickened.

Nutritional Information (per serving):

- Calories: 292.5
- Protein: 9g
- Sodium: 103.5mg
- Potassium: 609.5mg
- Carbohydrates: 61.5g

Berrylicious Smoothie

Prep Time: 5 minutes Cooking Time: Not applicable Serving Size: 1 serving

Ingredients:

- ⅛ cup cranberry juice cocktail
- ⅓ cup silken tofu, firm
- ¼ cup raspberries, frozen, unsweetened
- ¼ cup blueberries, frozen, unsweetened
- ½ tsp vanilla extract
- ¼ tsp powdered lemonade, such as Country Time

Instructions:

1. Pour the cranberry juice into a blender.
2. Add the silken tofu, frozen raspberries, frozen blueberries, vanilla extract, and powdered lemonade to the blender.
3. Blend until the mixture is very smooth.
4. Serve immediately and enjoy the berry goodness.

Nutritional Information (per serving):

- Calories: 115.5
- Protein: 6g
- Sodium: 14.5mg
- Potassium: 223.5mg
- Total Fat: 3g
- Carbohydrates: 18.5g
- Fiber: 1g

Blueberry Lemon Pound Cake

Preparation Time: 30 minutes Cooking Time: 45 minutes Serving Size: 1 slice

Ingredients:

- ½ cup non-fat cottage cheese
- ½ cup unsalted butter
- 3 fresh eggs
- 1 cup fat-free lemon yogurt
- 2 tsp vanilla extract
- ¼ cup Splenda
- 1¼ cups all-purpose flour
- ½ cup whole wheat flour
- 1 tsp baking powder
- ½ tsp baking soda
- ¼ tsp salt
- 2 tsp lemon zest
- 1 cup blueberries

Instructions:

1. Puree the cottage cheese until smooth.
2. In a mixer, combine the cottage cheese puree, butter, and Splenda. Beat until smooth.
3. Add eggs, yogurt, vanilla, lemon juice, and lemon zest to the mixture. Blend until smooth.
4. Sift together the all-purpose flour, whole wheat flour, baking powder, baking soda, and salt. Add to the mixing bowl and blend until smooth.
5. Gently fold in the blueberries.
6. Pour the batter into a greased 8" angel food cake pan.
7. Bake at 375°F for 35-40 minutes.

Nutritional Information Per Serving:

- Calories: 176.5
- Protein: 5.4g
- Sodium: 202.5mg
- Potassium: 106.2mg
- Total Fat: 9.4g
- Saturated Fat: 5.3g
- Cholesterol: 0mg
- Carbohydrates: 18.2g
- Fiber: 1.3g

Chicken and Zucchini Quiche

Preparation Time: 40 minutes Cooking Time: 1 hour Serving Size: 1/8 of the quiche

Ingredients:

- 9-inch pie crust, uncooked
- 6 oz. ground chicken
- 1½ zucchinis (6 oz.), diced
- 2 tsp ground sage
- ½ tsp onion powder
- 5 eggs
- 1 cup rice milk
- 1 tbsp poultry seasoning
- 3 slices of Swiss cheese

Instructions:

1. Preheat the oven to 350°F.
2. Line a pie plate with the pie dough.
3. In a sauté pan over medium heat, cook the ground chicken and zucchini with sage and onion powder until the chicken is thoroughly cooked. Let it cool to room temperature.

4. In a mixing bowl, whisk together eggs, rice milk, and poultry seasoning.

5. Place the cooled chicken and zucchini mixture into the bottom of the pie crust. Pour the egg mixture over the top.

6. Cut the cheese slices in half and arrange them on top of the egg mixture.

7. Bake on the lowest oven rack for 50 to 60 minutes, until the edges are browned and the center is firm.

Nutritional Information Per Serving:

- Calories: 187.5
- Protein: 10g
- Sodium: 134.5mg
- Potassium: 218.5mg
- Total Fat: 10.9g
- Saturated Fat: 4.3g
- Cholesterol: 0mg
- Carbohydrates: 12.2g
- Fiber: 0.6g

Cranberry Ginger Apricot Chutney

Preparation Time: 30 minutes Cooking Time: 45 minutes Serving Size: ¼ cup

Ingredients:

- 1 cup red onion, diced
- 1 tsp vegetable oil
- 1 tbsp grated ginger
- 1 cup apple, finely chopped (with skin)
- 1 tsp whole black peppercorn
- 10 oz (2 cups) cranberries, fresh or frozen
- 2 tbsp apple cider vinegar
- 2 tbsp apricot jam
- 1 tbsp lime juice
- Lime zest, for garnish

Instructions:

1. Heat the vegetable oil in a large skillet over medium-high heat.

2. Add the red onions and cook until soft, about 8-10 minutes.

3. Mix in the grated ginger, diced apple, and black peppercorns, cooking until the apples soften, about 5 minutes.

4. Add the cranberries, apple cider vinegar, apricot jam, and lime juice. Cook until the mixture thickens into a sauce-like consistency, about 15-20 minutes.

5. Garnish with lime zest before serving. Can be stored in the refrigerator for up to a week.

Nutritional Information Per Serving:

- Calories: 50.5
- Protein: 0.5g
- Sodium: 3.5mg
- Potassium: 93.5mg
- Total Fat: 0.7g
- Saturated Fat: 0.1g
- Cholesterol: 0mg
- Carbohydrates: 11.4g
- Fiber: 1.7

Fruit Crisp

Preparation Time: 30 minutes Cooking Time: 30 minutes Serving Size: 1 serving

Ingredients:

- 1 can (21 ounces) peaches in juice, drained
- 1 tsp lemon juice
- ½ cup brown sugar
- ¼ cup white flour
- ¾ cup oats
- ½ tsp cinnamon
- ½ tsp nutmeg
- ¼ stick cold unsalted butter

Instructions:

1. Preheat the oven to 350°F.
2. In a buttered muffin tin, place the drained peaches and sprinkle with lemon juice.
3. Mix brown sugar, flour, oats, cinnamon, and nutmeg in a bowl.
4. Cut in the butter until the mixture resembles wet sand.
5. Sprinkle this mixture over the peaches.
6. Bake for 25-30 minutes until the topping is browned and the filling is bubbly.
7. Serve warm.

Nutritional Information Per Serving:

- Calories: 309.5
- Protein: 3.9g
- Sodium: 15.1mg
- Potassium: 295.6mg
- Total Fat: 7g
- Saturated Fat: 3.8g
- Cholesterol: 0mg
- Carbohydrates: 60.9g
- Fiber: 3.9g

Grilled Low-Salt Flatbread

Prep Time: 20 minutes Cooking Time: 60 minutes Serving Size: 1 piece

Ingredients:

- 1 packet of active dry yeast
- 1/4 cup of lukewarm water
- 3/4 cup rice milk, warmed
- 2 tbsp granulated sugar
- 2 tbsp canola oil
- 3 to 3.5 cups of all-purpose flour

Instructions:

1. Begin by dissolving the yeast in the lukewarm water and set aside.
2. Warm the rice milk slightly, then combine it with the sugar and oil, cooling it until it's just warm to the touch.
3. In a large mixing bowl, start with 1.5 cups of flour. Add in the yeast mixture, stirring to combine.
4. Gradually mix in enough of the remaining flour to form a soft dough.
5. On a lightly floured surface, knead the dough for about 8 minutes, until it's smooth and elastic.
6. Place the dough in a bowl lightly coated with oil, covering it with plastic wrap. Let it rise in a warm spot until it doubles

in size, which may take 30 to 45 minutes due to the low salt content.

7. Once risen, punch down the dough to release air bubbles, then form it into flat disks, about 6 to 8 inches in diameter.

8. Prepare your grill by placing foil over it and lightly oiling the foil. Preheat the grill to a medium heat or until it reaches 350°F.

9. After heating, turn off the grill and place the dough disks on the foil. Grill each side until golden brown, which should take about 3 to 4 minutes per side.

10. Remove from the grill and add your favorite toppings before serving.

Nutritional Information Per Serving:

- Calories: 216.5
- Protein: 5.9g
- Sodium: 9.7mg
- Potassium: 62.5mg
- Total Fat: 4.6g
- Saturated Fat: 0.3g
- Cholesterol: 0mg
- Carbohydrates: 38.2g
- Fiber: 2.4g

Love Your Kidneys Breakfast Cereal

Prep Time: 10 minutes Cooking Time: 6 minutes Serving Size: 1/2 cup

Ingredients:

- 1 cup of Bulgur wheat
- 1 cup of Cranberry-Energy drink (Cranergy or similar)
- 1 tbsp granulated sugar
- 1 tbsp ground cinnamon
- 1/2 cup dried cranberries (Craisins)
- 1/4 cup almonds, finely chopped

Instructions:

1. In a microwave-safe bowl, combine the Bulgur wheat, Cranberry-Energy drink, sugar, and cinnamon. Stir these ingredients until they are well mixed.

2. Cover the bowl with a microwave-safe lid or plastic wrap. Microwave on high for 5 minutes, or until the liquid is fully absorbed by the Bulgur.

3. Once cooked, remove the bowl from the microwave. Carefully uncover and stir in the dried cranberries.

4. Garnish the top of the cereal with the chopped almonds, distributing them evenly.

Nutritional Information Per Serving:

- Calories: 250.5
- Protein: 6.6g
- Sodium: 14.6mg
- Potassium: 221.8mg

- Total Fat: 5.3g
- Saturated Fat: 0.4g
- Cholesterol: 0mg
- Carbohydrates: 51.3g
- Fiber: 8g

Peanut Butter Oatmeal

Prep Time: 10 minutes Cooking Time: 10 minutes Serving Size: 2/3 cup

Ingredients:

- 1 and 1/3 cups of raw oatmeal
- 4 tbsp of creamy peanut butter
- 1/4 cup of natural honey

Instructions:

1. Prepare the oatmeal according to the package instructions, making sure to skip adding any salt to the water.
2. Once the oatmeal is cooked and still warm, distribute it evenly into four serving bowls.
3. Add a generous tablespoon of creamy peanut butter and a tablespoon of honey to each bowl, swirling them into the oatmeal to combine the flavors beautifully.

Nutritional Information Per Serving:

- Calories: 238.5
- Protein: 6.5g
- Sodium: 71.5mg
- Potassium: 174.5mg
- Total Fat: 10.5g
- Saturated Fat: 2g
- Cholesterol: 0mg

- Carbohydrates: 35.5g
- Fiber: 3.5g

Pumpkin Pancakes

Prep Time: 20 minutes Cooking Time: 20 minutes Serving Size: 2 3-inch pancakes

Ingredients:

- 1 and 1/4 cups of all-purpose flour
- 1 tablespoon of brown sugar
- 3 packets of Stevia
- 1 teaspoon of baking powder
- 2 teaspoons of pumpkin pie spice
- 2 cups of salt-free Pumpkin Puree
- 2 cups of rice milk
- 2 egg whites

Instructions:

1. Combine the flour, brown sugar, Stevia, baking powder, and pumpkin pie spice in a mixing bowl.
2. In a different bowl, blend the pumpkin puree with rice milk until well mixed.
3. Beat the egg whites until soft peaks form.
4. Gradually mix the dry ingredients into the pumpkin and milk mixture until fully incorporated. Then, gently fold in the whipped egg whites.
5. Cook the pancakes on a medium-heated, lightly oiled griddle. Flip them when bubbles appear on the surface, and cook until the other side is golden brown.

Nutritional Information per Serving:

- Calories: 183.5

- Carbohydrates: 39.5g
- Dietary Fiber: 4.5g
- Protein: 5.9g
- Fat: 1.7g
- Saturated Fat: 0.7g
- Sodium: 130.5mg
- Potassium: 230.5mg
- Calcium: 177.5mg
- Phosphorus: 126.5mg

Pumpkin Cream Cheese Muffins

Prep Time: 25 minutes Cooking Time: 30 minutes Serving Size: 1 muffin

Ingredients:

- 8 ounces of cream cheese
- 3 large eggs
- 3 tablespoons of Stevia
- 1 and 3/4 cups of granulated sugar
- 2 cups of all-purpose flour
- 1 tablespoon of ground cinnamon
- 2 teaspoons of baking powder
- 1/4 teaspoon of baking soda
- 1 and 1/4 cups of pumpkin puree
- 1/3 cup of unsweetened apple sauce
- 2 teaspoons of pure vanilla extract

Instructions:

1. Preheat your oven to 375°F (190°C). Line muffin tins with paper liners.
2. In a small bowl, blend the cream cheese with one egg and Stevia until smooth. Set aside.
3. In a larger bowl, whisk together the remaining two eggs, pumpkin puree, apple sauce, and vanilla extract until well combined.
4. Sift together the sugar, flour, cinnamon, baking powder, and baking soda in another bowl.
5. Gradually add the dry ingredients to the pumpkin mixture, stirring just until the batter is moistened.
6. Fill each muffin cup halfway with the batter. Add a spoonful of the cream cheese mixture to the center of each, then cover with the remaining batter.
7. Bake in the preheated oven for 20 to 25 minutes, or until a toothpick inserted into the center of a muffin comes out clean.

Nutritional Information Per Serving:

- Calories: 145.5
- Carbohydrates: 25.5g
- Dietary Fiber: 1.4g
- Protein: 3g
- Fat: 4.5g
- Saturated Fat: 2.6g
- Sodium: 78.5mg
- Potassium: 62.5mg
- Phosphorus: 44.5mg
- Calcium: 43.5mg

Turkey Bacon, Egg, and Cheese Deviled Eggs

Prep Time: 35 minutes Cooking Time: 15 minutes Serving Size: 1 deviled egg

Ingredients:

- 6 large eggs
- 1/8 teaspoon of ground black pepper
- 2 slices of fully cooked turkey bacon
- 2 tablespoons of finely chopped spring onions or scallions
- 1 tablespoon of mustard
- 3 tablespoons of light mayonnaise
- 1 tablespoon of reduced-fat shredded sharp cheddar cheese

Instructions:

1. Arrange eggs in a single layer in a saucepan and cover with water. Bring to a rolling boil, then turn off the heat and let the eggs sit covered for 15 minutes.
2. Drain the hot water and cool the eggs in ice water. Once cooled, crack and peel the eggs.
3. Slice the eggs in half lengthwise. Gently remove the yolks and place them in a mixing bowl.
4. To the yolks, add the light mayonnaise, mustard, shredded cheese, one slice of crumbled turkey bacon, and black pepper. Mix until smooth and creamy.
5. Carefully spoon or pipe the yolk mixture back into the egg whites.
6. Crumble the remaining slice of turkey bacon and sprinkle it over the eggs, along with some extra cheese and chopped spring onions for garnish.

Nutritional Information Per Serving:

- Calories: 116.5
- Carbohydrates: 2.4g
- Dietary Fiber: 0.6g
- Protein: 8.6g
- Fat: 8.8g
- Saturated Fat: 2.7g
- Sodium: 255.9mg
- Potassium: 106.6mg
- Calcium: 44mg
- Phosphorus: 121.2mg

Lemon-Blueberry Corn Muffins

Prep Time: 15 minutes Cooking Time: 20 minutes Serving Size: 1 muffin

Ingredients:

- 1 cup fine cornmeal
- 3/4 cup whole wheat pastry flour
- 1/4 cup honey
- 2 tsp baking powder (low sodium)
- 1/2 tsp baking soda
- A pinch of salt (optional, can be omitted for a lower sodium version)
- Zest of 1 lemon
- 1 cup fresh blueberries
- 1 cup low-fat buttermilk
- 1/4 cup unsweetened applesauce
- 2 large eggs
- 1 tsp vanilla extract

Instructions:

1. Preheat your oven to 375°F (190°C). Line a muffin tin with paper liners or lightly grease with cooking spray.
2. In a large mixing bowl, whisk together the cornmeal, whole wheat pastry flour, baking powder, baking soda, and salt (if using). Stir in the lemon zest to evenly distribute.
3. In a separate bowl, beat the eggs lightly. Add the buttermilk, applesauce, honey, and vanilla extract, mixing until well combined.
4. Make a well in the center of the dry ingredients and pour in the wet ingredients. Stir just until the mixture is combined, being careful not to overmix. Gently fold in the blueberries.
5. Spoon the batter into the prepared muffin tin, filling each cup about three-quarters full.
6. Bake in the preheated oven for 20 minutes, or until a toothpick inserted into the center of a muffin comes out clean.
7. Allow the muffins to cool in the pan for 5 minutes before transferring them to a wire rack to cool completely.

Nutritional Information (per serving):

- Calories: 150
- Protein: 4g
- Sodium: 95mg (without added salt)
- Potassium: 125mg
- Total Fat: 2g
- Saturated Fat: 0.5g
- Cholesterol: 31mg
- Carbohydrates: 28g
- Fiber: 3g
- Sugars: 10g

Blueberry Oatmeal

Prep Time: 10 minutes Cooking Time: 5 minutes Serving Size: 1 cup

Ingredients:

- 1/2 cup rolled oats
- 1 cup water or low potassium milk alternative (e.g., almond milk)
- 1/2 tsp cinnamon
- 1/4 cup fresh blueberries
- 1 tbsp honey or maple syrup
- 1 tbsp ground flaxseed (optional)

Instructions:

1. In a small saucepan, bring water or milk alternative to a boil. Add oats and cinnamon, reducing heat to a simmer.
2. Cook for about 5 minutes, stirring occasionally, until the oats are soft and have absorbed most of the liquid.
3. Remove from heat and stir in the honey or maple syrup.
4. Serve in a bowl topped with fresh blueberries and a sprinkle of ground flaxseed for added fiber.

Nutritional Information (per serving):

- Calories: 215
- Protein: 6g
- Sodium: 30mg

- Potassium: 150mg
- Total Fat: 3.5g
- Saturated Fat: 0.5g
- Cholesterol: 0mg
- Carbohydrates: 42g
- Fiber: 6g

Blueberry Squares

Prep Time: 20 minutes Cooking Time: 25 minutes Serving Size: 1 square

Ingredients:

- 1 cup all-purpose flour
- 1/2 cup white sugar
- 1/4 tsp baking powder (low sodium)
- 1/2 cup unsalted butter, softened
- 1 egg, beaten
- 2 cups fresh blueberries
- 2 tbsp white sugar
- 1/2 tsp vanilla extract
- 1 tsp cornstarch dissolved in 1 tablespoon water

Instructions:

1. Preheat oven to 350°F. Grease a 9x9 inch baking pan.
2. In a medium bowl, combine flour, 1/2 cup sugar, baking powder, and butter until crumbly. Mix in beaten egg. Pat half of the mixture into the prepared pan.
3. In a separate bowl, mix blueberries, 2 tablespoons sugar, vanilla, and cornstarch mixture. Spread the blueberry mixture over the crust in the pan. Crumble remaining dough over the berry layer.
4. Bake for 25 minutes or until top is slightly brown. Cool completely before cutting into squares.

Nutritional Information (per serving):

- Calories: 165
- Protein: 2g
- Sodium: 15mg
- Potassium: 55mg
- Total Fat: 7g
- Saturated Fat: 4.5g
- Cholesterol: 31mg
- Carbohydrates: 24g
- Fiber: 1g

Bran Breakfast Bars

Prep Time: 15 minutes Cooking Time: 25 minutes Serving Size: 1 bar

Ingredients:

- 1 cup wheat bran
- 1/2 cup all-purpose flour
- 1/4 cup brown sugar
- 1/4 tsp low sodium baking powder
- 1/4 cup unsweetened applesauce
- 1 egg
- 1/4 cup low potassium milk alternative (e.g., almond milk)
- 1/2 tsp vanilla extract
- 1/4 cup raisins (optional)

Instructions:

1. Preheat oven to 350°F. Line an 8x8 inch baking pan with parchment paper.

2. In a large bowl, mix together wheat bran, flour, brown sugar, and baking powder.

3. Stir in applesauce, egg, milk alternative, and vanilla until well combined. Fold in raisins, if using.

4. Spread the mixture evenly in the prepared pan. Bake for 25 minutes or until set and edges are lightly browned.

5. Cool in the pan before cutting into bars.

Nutritional Information (per serving):

- Calories: 100
- Protein: 3g
- Sodium: 25mg
- Potassium: 120mg
- Total Fat: 1g
- Saturated Fat: 0g
- Cholesterol: 20mg
- Carbohydrates: 22g
- Fiber: 4g

LUNCH

Apple Rice Salad

Prep Time: 25 minutes

Cooking Time: 30 minutes

Serving Size: 1 cup

Ingredients:

- 1 cup brown rice, uncooked
- 2 cups water
- 1/4 tsp salt
- 1 large apple, diced
- 1/4 cup dried cranberries
- 1/4 cup chopped walnuts
- 2 tbsp apple cider vinegar
- 1 tbsp olive oil
- 1/2 tsp black pepper

Instructions:

1. Rinse brown rice under cold water until the water runs clear.
2. In a saucepan, bring water to a boil. Add rice and salt, reduce heat to low, cover, and cook for 30 minutes.
3. Remove from heat and let it stand covered for 5 minutes. Fluff with a fork and allow to cool.
4. In a large bowl, combine cooled rice with diced apple, cranberries, and walnuts.
5. In a small bowl, whisk together apple cider vinegar, olive oil, and black pepper.
6. Pour dressing over the rice mixture and toss to coat evenly.

Nutritional Information (per serving):

- Calories: 210
- Protein: 3g
- Sodium: 80mg
- Potassium: 150mg
- Total Fat: 7g
- Saturated Fat: 0.5g
- Cholesterol: 0mg
- Carbohydrates: 37g
- Fiber: 4g

Baked Macaroni and Cheese

- Prep Time: 15 minutes
- Cooking Time: 20 minutes
- Serving Size: 1/2 cup

Ingredients:

- 1 cup elbow macaroni, whole grain
- 2 cups water
- 1/4 tsp salt
- 1/2 cup shredded cheddar cheese, low sodium
- 1/4 cup milk, skimmed
- 1 tbsp flour, all-purpose
- 1/4 tsp paprika

Instructions:

1. Preheat oven to 350°F.
2. Cook macaroni according to package instructions until al dente; drain well.

3. In a saucepan over medium heat, whisk flour into milk until no lumps remain.

4. Add cheese and stir until melted. Season with salt and paprika.

5. Combine cheese sauce with cooked macaroni and transfer to a baking dish.

6. Bake for 20 minutes or until the top is golden brown.

Nutritional Information (per serving):

- Calories: 220
- Protein: 10g
- Sodium: 150mg
- Potassium: 100mg
- Total Fat: 6g
- Saturated Fat: 3g
- Cholesterol: 15mg
- Carbohydrates: 30g
- Fiber: 2g

Baked Potato Soup

Prep Time: 10 minutes

Cooking Time: 35 minutes

Serving Size: 1 cup

Ingredients:

- 2 large potatoes, peeled and diced
- 3 cups water
- 1/4 tsp salt
- 1/4 cup onion, chopped
- 1/2 cup milk, skimmed
- 1/4 tsp black pepper
- 1/4 cup sour cream, low-fat
- 1 tbsp chives, chopped

Instructions:

1. In a large pot, bring potatoes, water, and salt to a boil. Reduce heat and simmer until potatoes are tender.

2. Remove half of the potatoes and set aside. Blend the remaining soup until smooth.

3. Return the reserved potatoes to the pot. Add onion, milk, and black pepper.

4. Cook over low heat for 5 minutes. Stir in sour cream and heat through without boiling.

5. Serve hot, garnished with chives.

Nutritional Information (per serving):

- Calories: 150
- Protein: 4g
- Sodium: 125mg
- Potassium: 470mg
- Total Fat: 2g
- Saturated Fat: 1g
- Cholesterol: 5mg
- Carbohydrates: 28g
- Fiber: 3g

Beef Barley Soup

Prep Time: 15 minutes

Cooking Time: 1 hour

Serving Size: 1 cup

Ingredients:

- 1/2 lb beef stew meat, trimmed and cubed
- 6 cups water
- 1/4 tsp salt
- 1/2 cup barley, uncooked
- 1 cup carrots, diced
- 1/2 cup celery, diced
- 1/4 cup onion, chopped

Instructions:

1. In a large pot, brown beef over medium heat.
2. Add water and salt; bring to a boil. Reduce heat to low and simmer for about an hour.
3. Add barley, carrots, celery, and onion to the pot. Simmer for another 30 minutes or until vegetables are tender.

Nutritional Information (per serving):

- Calories: 180
- Protein: 14g
- Sodium: 55mg
- Potassium: 300mg
- Total Fat: 4g
- Saturated Fat: 1.5g
- Cholesterol: 35mg
- Carbohydrates: 20g
- Fiber: 4g

Canned Fish Tacos

Prep Time: 15 minutes

Cooking Time: 10 minutes

Serving Size: 2 tacos

Ingredients:

- 1 can (6 oz) low-sodium canned tuna or salmon, drained
- 4 small corn tortillas
- 1/2 cup red cabbage, shredded
- 1/4 cup Greek yogurt, plain
- 1 tbsp lime juice
- 1/2 tsp cumin
- 1/2 tsp paprika
- Fresh cilantro, chopped (optional)

Instructions:

1. In a bowl, mix together Greek yogurt, lime juice, cumin, and paprika.
2. Warm the corn tortillas in a pan over medium heat for about 30 seconds on each side.
3. Place the canned fish onto the tortillas.
4. Top with shredded cabbage and a dollop of the Greek yogurt mixture.
5. Garnish with cilantro if desired.

Nutritional Information (per serving):

- Calories: Approx. 200
- Protein: 20g
- Sodium: Less than 200mg
- Potassium: Approx. 300mg
- Total Fat: 5g
- Saturated Fat: 1g
- Cholesterol: 30mg
- Carbohydrates: 18g

- Fiber: 3g

Chicken and Corn Chowder

Prep Time: 20 minutes

Cooking Time: 25 minutes

Serving Size: 1 cup

Ingredients:

- 1/2 lb chicken breast, skinless and boneless, cubed
- 2 cups low-sodium chicken broth
- 1 cup corn kernels, fresh or frozen
- 1/2 cup carrots, diced
- 1/2 cup celery, diced
- 1/4 cup onion, chopped
- 1 garlic clove, minced
- 1/2 cup milk, low-fat
- 2 tbsp all-purpose flour
- Salt-free seasoning blend to taste

Instructions:

1. In a large pot, sauté onion and garlic until translucent.
2. Add chicken cubes and cook until no longer pink.
3. Stir in carrots and celery; cook for another few minutes.
4. Sprinkle flour over the vegetables and chicken; stir well.
5. Gradually pour in chicken broth while stirring constantly to avoid lumps.
6. Add corn kernels and bring to a simmer.
7. Reduce heat and let simmer for about 15 minutes or until vegetables are tender.
8. Stir in milk and heat through without boiling.
9. Season with salt-free seasoning blend.

Nutritional Information (per serving):

- Calories: Approx. 150
- Protein: 14g
- Sodium: Less than 200mg
- Potassium: Approx. 350mg
- Total Fat: 3g
- Saturated Fat: 0.5g
- Cholesterol: 25mg
- Carbohydrates: 15g
- Fiber: 2g

Chicken and Dumplings

Prep Time: 30 minutes

Cooking Time: 45 minutes

Serving Size: 2 dumplings

Ingredients:

- 1/2 lb chicken breast, skinless and boneless, cubed
- 4 cups low-sodium chicken broth
- 1 cup carrots, sliced
- 1/2 cup celery, sliced
- 1/4 cup onion, chopped
- 1 garlic clove, minced
- 1 cup all-purpose flour
- 2 tsp baking powder
- 1/2 cup milk, low-fat
- Salt-free seasoning blend to taste

Instructions:

1. In a large pot, sauté onion and garlic until translucent.

2. Add chicken cubes and cook until no longer pink.

3. Stir in carrots and celery; cook for another few minutes.

4. Pour in chicken broth and bring to a simmer.

5. In a mixing bowl, combine flour, baking powder, and a pinch of salt-free seasoning blend.

6. Gradually add milk to the dry ingredients, stirring until a soft dough forms.

7. Drop spoonfuls of dough into the simmering soup.

8. Cover and let simmer for about 15 minutes or until dumplings are cooked through.

Nutritional Information (per serving):

- Calories: Approx. 250
- Protein: 22g
- Sodium: Less than 200mg
- Potassium: Approx. 400mg
- Total Fat: 4g
- Saturated Fat: 1g
- Cholesterol: 45mg
- Carbohydrates: 25g
- Fiber: 2g

Chicken N' Orange Salad Sandwich

Prep Time: 15 minutes

Cooking Time: None

Serving Size: 1 sandwich

Ingredients:

- 1/2 lb chicken breast, cooked and shredded
- 1/4 cup Greek yogurt, plain
- 2 tbsp orange juice
- Zest of one orange
- Salt-free seasoning blend to taste
- Lettuce leaves
- Whole wheat bread slices

Instructions:

1. In a bowl, mix together shredded chicken, Greek yogurt, orange juice, orange zest, and salt-free seasoning blend.

2. Place lettuce leaves on one slice of bread.

3. Spread the chicken mixture over the lettuce.

4. Top with another slice of bread.

Nutritional Information (per serving):

- Calories: Approx. 300
- Protein: 28g
- Sodium: Less than 200mg
- Potassium: Approx. 350mg
- Total Fat: 6g
- Saturated Fat: 1g
- Cholesterol: 50mg

- Carbohydrates: 32g
- Fiber: 5g

Chinese Chicken Salad

Prep Time: 20 minutes

Cooking Time: None

Serving Size: 1 bowl

Ingredients:

- 1/2 lb chicken breast, cooked and shredded
- 3 cups mixed greens (lettuce, spinach)
- 1/2 cup red bell pepper, sliced
- 1/4 cup carrot, shredded

• Dressing:

- 3 tbsp rice vinegar
- 1 tbsp sesame oil
- Salt-free seasoning blend to taste

Instructions:

1. In a large bowl, combine mixed greens, red bell pepper slices, shredded carrot, and shredded chicken.
2. In a small bowl, whisk together rice vinegar, sesame oil, and salt-free seasoning blend for the dressing.
3. Drizzle dressing over the salad just before serving.

Nutritional Information (per serving):

- Calories: Approx. 250
- Protein: 26g
- Sodium: Less than 200mg
- Potassium: Approx. 400mg
- Total Fat: 8g
- Saturated Fat: 1g

- Cholesterol: None
- Carbohydrates: 12g
- Fiber: 3g

Cider Cream Chicken

Prep Time: 25 minutes

Cooking Time: 30 minutes

Serving Size: 1 portion

Ingredients:

- 2 boneless, skinless chicken breasts
- 1 tbsp olive oil
- 1/2 cup apple cider
- 1/4 cup low sodium chicken broth
- 1/4 cup heavy cream
- 1 tbsp Dijon mustard
- 1 tsp fresh thyme leaves
- Salt and pepper to taste

Instructions:

1. Season the chicken breasts with salt and pepper.
2. Heat olive oil in a skillet over medium heat and cook the chicken until golden brown on both sides.
3. Remove the chicken and set aside. In the same skillet, add apple cider and chicken broth, bring to a simmer.
4. Stir in heavy cream, Dijon mustard, and thyme leaves. Return the chicken to the skillet.
5. Cook until the chicken is done and the sauce has thickened.
6. Adjust seasoning if necessary and serve hot.

Nutritional Information (per serving):

- Calories: Approximately 300
- Protein: 27g
- Sodium: Less than 200mg
- Potassium: Less than 500mg
- Total Fat: 15g
- Saturated Fat: 5g
- Cholesterol: Less than 100mg
- Carbohydrates: 8g
- Fiber: Less than 1g

Cowboy Caviar Bean and Rice Salad

Prep Time: 15 minutes

Cooking Time: No cooking required

Serving Size: 1 cup

Ingredients:

- 1 cup cooked brown rice, cooled
- 1/2 cup black beans, rinsed and drained
- 1/2 cup corn kernels, fresh or frozen (thawed)
- 1/4 cup red bell pepper, diced
- 2 tbsp red onion, finely chopped
- 2 tbsp cilantro, chopped
- Juice of one lime
- Salt and pepper to taste

Instructions:

1. In a large bowl, combine brown rice, black beans, corn kernels, red bell pepper, red onion, and cilantro.
2. Squeeze lime juice over the mixture and season with salt and pepper.
3. Toss everything together until well mixed.
4. Serve chilled or at room temperature.

Nutritional Information (per serving):

- Calories: Approximately 150
- Protein: 5g
- Sodium: Less than 200mg
- Potassium: Less than 300mg
- Total Fat: Less than 1g
- Saturated Fat: 0g
- Cholesterol: 0mg
- Carbohydrates: 30g
- Fiber: 5g

Creamy Tuna Twist

Prep Time: 15 minutes

Cooking Time: No cooking required

Serving Size: 1 cup

Ingredients:

- 1 can (5 oz) low-sodium tuna, drained
- 1/2 cup whole grain pasta, cooked and cooled
- 1/4 cup celery, diced
- 1/4 cup apple, diced
- 2 tbsp plain Greek yogurt
- 1 tbsp lemon juice
- 1 tsp dried dill weed
- Salt and pepper to taste

Instructions:

1. In a bowl, flake the tuna with a fork.
2. Add cooked pasta, celery, and apple to the tuna.

3. In a separate small bowl, mix Greek yogurt, lemon juice, and dill weed.

4. Combine the yogurt dressing with the tuna mixture.

5. Season with salt and pepper to taste.

6. Serve chilled or at room temperature.

Nutritional Information (per serving):

- Calories: Approximately 200
- Protein: 20g
- Sodium: Less than 200mg
- Potassium: Less than 300mg
- Total Fat: 3g
- Saturated Fat: Less than 1g
- Cholesterol: Less than 30mg
- Carbohydrates: 20g
- Fiber: 3g

Curry Chicken Salad

Prep Time: 20 minutes

Cooking Time: No cooking required

Serving Size: 1 cup

Ingredients:

- 2 cups cooked chicken breast, diced
- 1/4 cup plain Greek yogurt
- 1 tbsp curry powder
- 1/2 apple, diced
- 1/4 cup raisins
- Salt and pepper to taste

Instructions:

1. In a large bowl, combine diced chicken breast with Greek yogurt and curry powder.

2. Mix in diced apple and raisins.

3. Season with salt and pepper to taste.

4. Serve chilled or on a bed of lettuce.

Nutritional Information (per serving):

- Calories: Approximately 250
- Protein: 30g
- Sodium: Less than 200mg
- Potassium: Less than 400mg
- Total Fat: 5g
- Saturated Fat: Less than 1g
- Cholesterol: Less than 80mg
- Carbohydrates: 15g
- Fiber: 2g

Fruity Chicken Salad

Prep Time: 20 minutes

Cooking Time: No cooking required

Serving Size: 1 cup

Ingredients:

- 2 cups cooked chicken breast, shredded
- 1/4 cup grapes, halved
- 1/4 cup mandarin oranges, drained
- 1/4 cup plain Greek yogurt
- 1 tbsp honey
- 1 tsp poppy seeds
- Salt and pepper to taste

Instructions:

1. In a large bowl, combine shredded chicken, grapes, and mandarin oranges.

2. In a separate small bowl, whisk together Greek yogurt, honey, and poppy seeds.

3. Pour the dressing over the chicken mixture and toss to coat evenly.

4. Season with salt and pepper to taste.

5. Serve chilled or on a bed of mixed greens.

Nutritional Information (per serving):

- Calories: Approximately 220
- Protein: 25g
- Sodium: Less than 200mg
- Potassium: Less than 350mg
- Total Fat: 3g
- Saturated Fat: Less than 1g
- Cholesterol: Less than 70mg
- Carbohydrates: 20g
- Fiber: 2g

Green Tomatoes with Goat Cheese

Prep Time: 10 minutes

Cooking Time: No cooking required

Serving Size: 2 slices

Ingredients:

- 2 large green tomatoes, sliced thickly
- 1/4 cup goat cheese, crumbled
- 2 tbsp balsamic vinegar reduction
- Fresh basil leaves for garnish

Instructions:

- Arrange green tomato slices on a plate.
- Sprinkle crumbled goat cheese over the tomato slices.
- Drizzle balsamic vinegar reduction over the top.
- Garnish with fresh basil leaves before serving.

Nutritional Information (per serving):

- Calories: Approximately 90
- Protein: 4g
- Sodium: Less than 150mg
- Potassium: Less than 200mg
- Total Fat: 5g
- Saturated Fat: Less than 3g
- Cholesterol: Less than 10mg
- Carbohydrates: 6g
- Fiber: Less than 2g

Grilled Vegetable Pasta Salad

Prep Time: 20 minutes

Cooking Time: 10 minutes

Serving Size: 1 cup

Ingredients:

- 1 cup whole grain pasta, cooked and cooled
- 1/2 cup zucchini, sliced and grilled
- 1/2 cup bell peppers, assorted colors, sliced and grilled
- 1/4 cup cherry tomatoes, halved
- 2 tbsp red onion, finely chopped
- 1 tbsp olive oil
- 1 tbsp balsamic vinegar
- Salt and pepper to taste

Instructions:

1. In a large bowl, combine cooked pasta with grilled zucchini, bell peppers, cherry tomatoes, and red onion.
2. Drizzle olive oil and balsamic vinegar over the salad.
3. Toss everything together until well mixed.
4. Season with salt and pepper to taste.

5. Serve chilled or at room temperature.

Nutritional Information (per serving):

- Calories: Approximately 180
- Protein: 5g
- Sodium: Less than 200mg
- Potassium: Less than 300mg
- Total Fat: 5g
- Saturated Fat: Less than 1g
- Cholesterol: 0mg
- Carbohydrates: 30g
- Fiber: 5g

Herb Breaded Chicken

Prep Time: 15 minutes

Cooking Time: 25 minutes

Serving Size: 1 piece

Ingredients:

- 4 boneless, skinless chicken breasts
- 1/2 cup whole wheat breadcrumbs
- 2 tbsp Parmesan cheese, grated
- 1 tsp dried Italian herbs
- Salt and pepper to taste
- Olive oil spray

Instructions:

1. Preheat oven to 375°F.
2. In a shallow dish, combine breadcrumbs, Parmesan cheese, and dried herbs.
3. Season chicken breasts with salt and pepper.
4. Coat each chicken breast in the breadcrumb mixture.
5. Place breaded chicken on a baking sheet lined with parchment paper and lightly spray with olive oil.
6. Bake for 25 minutes or until chicken is cooked through.

Nutritional Information (per serving):

- Calories: Approximately 220
- Protein: 30g
- Sodium: Less than 300mg
- Potassium: Less than 400mg
- Total Fat: 5g
- Saturated Fat: Less than 2g
- Cholesterol: Less than 70mg
- Carbohydrates: 10g
- Fiber: Less than 1g

Irish Baked Potato Soup

Prep Time: 15 minutes Cooking Time: 30 minutes Serving Size: 1 cup

Ingredients:

- 4 large potatoes, peeled and diced
- 1 tablespoon unsalted butter
- 1/4 cup onion, finely chopped
- 2 cloves garlic, minced
- 4 cups low-sodium chicken or vegetable broth
- 1/2 cup carrots, diced
- 1/2 cup celery, diced
- 1/4 teaspoon ground black pepper
- 1 cup low-fat milk
- 2 tablespoons all-purpose flour
- 1/4 cup sour cream, low in sodium
- Chives, chopped for garnish

Instructions:

1. In a large pot, melt the butter over medium heat. Add the onion and garlic, sautéing until soft.

2. Add the broth, potatoes, carrots, celery, and black pepper. Bring to a boil, then reduce heat and simmer until vegetables are tender, about 20 minutes.

3. In a small bowl, whisk together the milk and flour until smooth. Gradually stir this mixture into the soup.

4. Continue cooking, stirring frequently, until the soup thickens, about 10 minutes.

5. Remove from heat. Stir in sour cream. Use an immersion blender to puree the soup to your desired consistency.

6. Serve hot, garnished with chives.

Nutritional Information (per serving):

- Calories: 210
- Protein: 6g
- Sodium: 190mg
- Potassium: 750mg
- Total Fat: 5g
- Saturated Fat: 3g
- Cholesterol: 15mg
- Carbohydrates: 35g
- Fiber: 3g

Kohlrabi Soup

Prep Time: 10 minutes Cooking Time: 25 minutes Serving Size: 1 cup

Ingredients:

- 2 medium kohlrabi bulbs, peeled and diced
- 1 tablespoon olive oil
- 1/4 cup onion, chopped
- 2 cups low-sodium vegetable broth
- 1/2 teaspoon dried thyme
- 1/4 teaspoon ground black pepper
- 1/2 cup unsweetened almond milk
- Lemon zest, for garnish

Instructions:

1. In a large pot, heat the olive oil over medium heat. Add the onion and sauté until translucent.

2. Add the kohlrabi, broth, thyme, and black pepper. Bring to a boil, then reduce heat and simmer until kohlrabi is tender, about 20 minutes.

3. Use an immersion blender to puree the soup until smooth.

4. Stir in the almond milk and heat through, but do not boil.

5. Serve hot, garnished with lemon zest.

Nutritional Information (per serving):

- Calories: 80
- Protein: 2g
- Sodium: 50mg
- Potassium: 290mg
- Total Fat: 3.5g
- Saturated Fat: 0.5g

- Cholesterol: 0mg
- Carbohydrates: 11g
- Fiber: 5g

Lemon Curry Chicken Salad

Prep Time: 20 minutes Cooking Time: 0 minutes Serving Size: 1/2 cup

Ingredients:

- 2 cups cooked chicken breast, diced
- 1/4 cup celery, diced
- 1/4 cup apple, diced
- 1/4 cup low-fat mayonnaise
- 1 tablespoon lemon juice
- 1/2 teaspoon curry powder
- Lettuce leaves, for serving

Instructions:

1. In a large bowl, combine the chicken, celery, and apple.
2. In a small bowl, mix together the mayonnaise, lemon juice, and curry powder. Stir into the chicken mixture until well coated.
3. Refrigerate for at least 1 hour to allow flavors to meld.
4. Serve on lettuce leaves.

Nutritional Information (per serving):

- Calories: 150
- Protein: 20g
- Sodium: 125mg
- Potassium: 220mg
- Total Fat: 4.5g
- Saturated Fat: 1g
- Cholesterol: 55mg

- Carbohydrates: 7g
- Fiber: 1g

Lentil Meatballs or Patties

Prep Time: 15 minutes Cooking Time: 20 minutes Serving Size: 2 meatballs or patties

Ingredients:

- 1 cup green lentils, cooked
- 1/4 cup onion, finely chopped
- 1 clove garlic, minced
- 1/4 cup carrots, grated
- 1/4 cup breadcrumbs, low sodium
- 1 egg, beaten
- 1 teaspoon dried oregano
- 1/4 teaspoon ground black pepper
- Olive oil, for cooking

Instructions:

1. Preheat your oven to 375°F (190°C). Line a baking sheet with parchment paper.
2. In a large bowl, mash the lentils. Mix in the onion, garlic, carrots, breadcrumbs, egg, oregano, and black pepper until well combined.
3. Form the mixture into meatballs or patties and place on the prepared baking sheet.
4. Brush lightly with olive oil and bake for 20 minutes, or until golden and firm.
5. Serve warm.

Nutritional Information (per serving):

- Calories: 190
- Protein: 12g

- Sodium: 70mg
- Potassium: 330mg
- Total Fat: 3g
- Saturated Fat: 0.5g

- Cholesterol: 53mg
- Carbohydrates: 30g
- Fiber: 9g

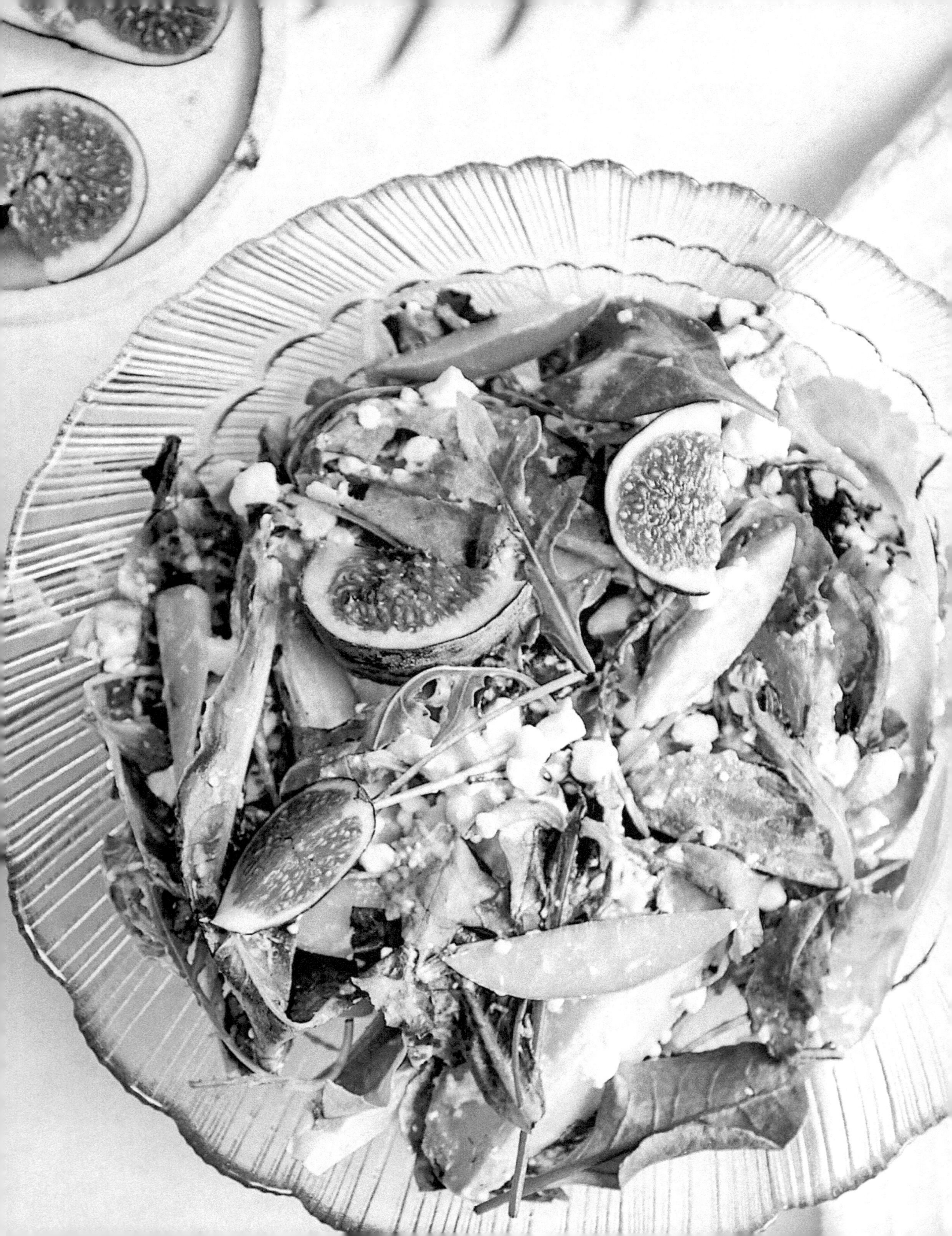

DINNER

Apple Almond Galette

Prep Time: 20 minutes Cooking Time: 25 minutes Serving Size: 1 slice

Ingredients:

- 1 1/2 cups all-purpose flour
- 1/4 cup almond flour
- 1/2 teaspoon salt
- 1/2 cup unsalted butter, chilled and diced
- 1/4 cup ice water
- 3 medium apples, peeled, cored, and thinly sliced
- 1 tablespoon lemon juice
- 2 tablespoons honey
- 1/2 teaspoon ground cinnamon
- 1 egg, beaten for egg wash
- 2 tablespoons sliced almonds

Instructions:

1. In a large bowl, mix together the all-purpose flour, almond flour, and salt. Cut in the butter until the mixture resembles coarse crumbs. Gradually add ice water, stirring until the dough comes together. Wrap in plastic and refrigerate for at least 30 minutes.
2. Preheat oven to 375°F. In a bowl, toss the sliced apples with lemon juice, honey, and cinnamon.
3. On a floured surface, roll out the dough into a 12-inch circle. Transfer to a baking sheet lined with parchment paper.
4. Arrange the apple slices over the dough, leaving a 2-inch border. Fold the edges over the apples, pleating as needed.
5. Brush the crust with egg wash and sprinkle with sliced almonds.
6. Bake for 25 minutes or until the crust is golden and the apples are tender.
7. Let cool before serving.

Nutritional Information (per serving):

- Calories: 220
- Protein: 3g
- Sodium: 75mg
- Potassium: 115mg
- Total Fat: 12g
- Saturated Fat: 6g
- Cholesterol: 40mg
- Carbohydrates: 26g
- Fiber: 2g

Apple Caramel Crisp

Prep Time: 15 minutes Cooking Time: 30 minutes Serving Size: 1/2 cup

Ingredients:

- 4 medium apples, peeled, cored, and sliced
- 1 tablespoon lemon juice
- 2 tablespoons brown sugar substitute
- 1 teaspoon ground cinnamon

- 1/2 cup rolled oats
- 1/4 cup almond flour
- 1/4 cup unsalted butter, melted
- 2 tablespoons sugar-free caramel syrup

Instructions:

1. Preheat oven to 350°F. Toss the apple slices with lemon juice, brown sugar substitute, and cinnamon in a baking dish.
2. In a bowl, combine rolled oats, almond flour, and melted butter until the mixture resembles coarse crumbs.
3. Sprinkle the oat mixture over the apples. Drizzle with sugar-free caramel syrup.
4. Bake for 30 minutes or until the topping is golden and the apples are tender.
5. Serve warm.

Nutritional Information (per serving):

- Calories: 180
- Protein: 2g
- Sodium: 25mg
- Potassium: 120mg
- Total Fat: 9g
- Saturated Fat: 4.5g
- Cholesterol: 20mg
- Carbohydrates: 24g
- Fiber: 3g

Apple Cranberry Walnut Salad

Prep Time: 10 minutes Cooking Time: 0 minutes Serving Size: 1 cup

Ingredients:

- 2 medium apples, diced
- 1/4 cup dried cranberries, low sugar
- 1/4 cup walnuts, chopped
- 1/4 cup celery, diced
- 2 tablespoons mayonnaise, low sodium
- 1 tablespoon lemon juice

Instructions:

1. In a large bowl, combine diced apples, dried cranberries, chopped walnuts, and diced celery.
2. In a small bowl, whisk together mayonnaise and lemon juice. Pour over the apple mixture and toss to coat evenly.
3. Chill in the refrigerator for at least 1 hour before serving.

Nutritional Information (per serving):

- Calories: 150
- Protein: 2g
- Sodium: 55mg
- Potassium: 95mg
- Total Fat: 9g
- Saturated Fat: 1g
- Cholesterol: 5mg
- Carbohydrates: 17g
- Fiber: 3g

Apple Sage Stuffing

Prep Time: 15 minutes Cooking Time: 25 minutes Serving Size: 1/2 cup

Ingredients:

- 4 cups bread cubes, low sodium
- 1 cup unsalted chicken broth
- 1 medium apple, diced
- 1/4 cup onion, finely chopped
- 1/4 cup celery, diced
- 1 tablespoon unsalted butter
- 1 teaspoon dried sage
- 1/4 teaspoon ground black pepper

Instructions:

1. Preheat oven to 350°F. In a large skillet, melt the butter over medium heat. Add onion and celery, cooking until soft.
2. Stir in the diced apple, sage, and black pepper. Cook for another 2 minutes.
3. In a large bowl, combine the bread cubes with the apple mixture. Gradually add chicken broth, tossing gently until moistened.
4. Transfer to a baking dish and cover with foil. Bake for 20 minutes, then remove foil and bake for an additional 5 minutes or until the top is crisp.
5. Serve warm.

Nutritional Information (per serving):

- Calories: 120
- Protein: 3g
- Sodium: 150mg
- Potassium: 90mg
- Total Fat: 3g
- Saturated Fat: 1.5g
- Cholesterol: 5mg
- Carbohydrates: 20g
- Fiber: 2g

Birthday Popcorn

Prep Time: 5 minutes Cooking Time: 5 minutes Serving Size: 1 cup

Ingredients:

- 1/2 cup popcorn kernels
- 1 tablespoon canola oil
- 1/4 teaspoon salt (optional, and to taste)
- 2 tablespoons melted unsalted butter (optional)
- 1 tablespoon nutritional yeast (for a cheesy flavor without the added phosphorus)
- 1/4 cup dried cranberries
- 1/4 cup sliced almonds

Instructions:

1. Heat the oil in a large pot over medium heat. Add the popcorn kernels and cover with a lid. Shake the pot occasionally until the popping slows down.
2. Once popped, remove from heat and transfer to a large bowl.
3. Drizzle with melted butter, if using, and sprinkle with salt and nutritional yeast. Toss well to coat evenly.
4. Add the dried cranberries and sliced almonds, and toss again until well mixed.

5. Serve immediately or store in an airtight container for later enjoyment.

Nutritional Information (per serving):

- Calories: 150
- Protein: 3g
- Sodium: 50mg (without added salt)
- Potassium: 75mg
- Total Fat: 8g
- Saturated Fat: 1.5g (without added butter)
- Cholesterol: 0mg
- Carbohydrates: 18g
- Fiber: 4g

Bolognese with Rice Noodles

Prep Time: 15 minutes Cooking Time: 30 minutes Serving Size: 1 cup

Ingredients:

- 1/2 pound lean ground beef (choose a low-fat variety to reduce phosphorus)
- 1 tablespoon olive oil
- 1/4 cup onion, finely chopped
- 1 clove garlic, minced
- 1 cup low-sodium tomato sauce
- 1/2 teaspoon dried oregano
- 1/2 teaspoon dried basil
- 1/4 teaspoon ground black pepper
- 8 ounces rice noodles

Instructions:

1. Heat the olive oil in a large skillet over medium heat. Add the onion and garlic, cooking until softened.
2. Add the ground beef, breaking it up with a spoon, and cook until browned.
3. Stir in the tomato sauce, oregano, basil, and black pepper. Simmer for 20 minutes, allowing the flavors to meld.
4. Meanwhile, cook the rice noodles according to the package instructions, then drain.
5. Serve the Bolognese sauce over the cooked rice noodles.

Nutritional Information (per serving):

- Calories: 320
- Protein: 14g
- Sodium: 100mg
- Potassium: 350mg
- Total Fat: 10g
- Saturated Fat: 3g
- Cholesterol: 35mg
- Carbohydrates: 44g
- Fiber: 2g

Bow-Tie Pasta Salad

Prep Time: 15 minutes Cooking Time: 10 minutes Serving Size: 1 cup

Ingredients:

- 8 ounces bow-tie pasta (use whole wheat if possible for added fiber)
- 1 cup cherry tomatoes, halved
- 1/2 cup cucumber, diced
- 1/4 cup red onion, finely sliced
- 1/4 cup low-sodium Italian dressing
- 1 tablespoon fresh basil, chopped
- 1 tablespoon fresh parsley, chopped

- Black pepper to taste

Instructions:

1. Cook the bow-tie pasta according to package instructions, then rinse under cold water and drain.

2. In a large bowl, combine the cooked pasta with cherry tomatoes, cucumber, and red onion.

3. Pour over the Italian dressing and toss to coat evenly.

4. Add the chopped basil, parsley, and black pepper. Toss again before serving.

Nutritional Information (per serving):

- Calories: 220
- Protein: 7g
- Sodium: 70mg
- Potassium: 150mg
- Total Fat: 4g
- Saturated Fat: 0.5g
- Cholesterol: 0mg
- Carbohydrates: 40g
- Fiber: 5g

Creamy Curry Rice & Apple Salad

Prep Time: 15 minutes Cooking Time: 25 minutes Serving Size: 1 cup Ingredients:

- 1 cup brown rice, uncooked
- 2 cups water
- 1/4 tsp salt (optional, can be omitted for a lower sodium option)
- 1 medium apple, diced
- 1/4 cup celery, finely chopped
- 1/4 cup red bell pepper, finely chopped
- 2 tbsp onion, finely chopped
- 1/2 cup plain, non-fat Greek yogurt
- 1 tbsp curry powder (adjust based on tolerance)
- 1 tsp honey
- 2 tbsp almond slivers, toasted

Instructions:

1. Rinse brown rice under cold water. Combine rice, water, and salt in a saucepan and bring to a boil. Reduce heat to low, cover, and simmer until water is absorbed and rice is tender, about 25 minutes.

2. Allow rice to cool slightly. In a large bowl, combine the cooked rice, diced apple, celery, red bell pepper, and onion.

3. In a separate small bowl, mix Greek yogurt, curry powder, and honey until well blended. Pour this dressing over the rice mixture and toss until everything is evenly coated.

4. Refrigerate the salad for at least an hour before serving. Garnish with toasted almond slivers before serving.

Nutritional Information (per serving):

- Calories: 150
- Protein: 4g
- Sodium: 75mg (without added salt)
- Potassium: 200mg
- Total Fat: 2g
- Saturated Fat: 0g
- Cholesterol: 0mg

- Carbohydrates: 28g
- Fiber: 3g

Favorite Cranberry Salad

Prep Time: 20 minutes Cooking Time: 0 minutes Serving Size: 1/2 cup

Ingredients:

- 1 cup fresh cranberries, finely chopped
- 1 cup pineapple, canned in juice, drained and chopped
- 1/4 cup sugar substitute (e.g., stevia blend)
- 1 cup celery, finely chopped
- 1/2 cup walnuts, chopped (optional, omit if phosphorus needs to be strictly controlled)
- 1 cup plain, non-fat Greek yogurt

Instructions:

1. Combine the chopped cranberries and sugar substitute in a bowl. Let it sit for 10 minutes to allow the cranberries to release their natural juices and sweeten.
2. Add the chopped pineapple, celery, and walnuts (if using) to the cranberries. Mix well.
3. Fold in the Greek yogurt until all ingredients are well combined.
4. Refrigerate for at least 2 hours before serving to allow flavors to meld.

Nutritional Information (per serving):

- Calories: 120
- Protein: 4g
- Sodium: 45mg
- Potassium: 180mg
- Total Fat: 5g (less without walnuts)
- Saturated Fat: 0g
- Cholesterol: 0mg
- Carbohydrates: 17g
- Fiber: 2g

Grilled Vegetables

Prep Time: 15 minutes Cooking Time: 20 minutes Serving Size: 1 cup

Ingredients:

- 1 medium zucchini, sliced into 1/2-inch thick rounds
- 1 yellow squash, sliced into 1/2-inch thick rounds
- 1 red bell pepper, seeded and cut into 1-inch pieces
- 1 tablespoon olive oil
- 1/4 teaspoon garlic powder
- 1/4 teaspoon onion powder
- 1/4 teaspoon dried oregano
- 1/4 teaspoon dried thyme
- Freshly ground black pepper, to taste

Instructions:

1. Preheat the grill to medium-high heat.
2. In a large bowl, toss the zucchini, yellow squash, and red bell pepper with olive oil, garlic powder, onion powder, oregano, thyme, and black pepper until well coated.
3. Arrange the vegetables in a single layer on a grill basket or directly on the grill grates. Grill for 10-12 minutes, turning

occasionally, until the vegetables are tender and have nice grill marks.

4. Remove the vegetables from the grill and serve immediately.

Nutritional Information (per serving):

- Calories: 60
- Protein: 1.5g
- Sodium: 20mg
- Potassium: 300mg
- Total Fat: 3.5g
- Saturated Fat: 0.5g
- Cholesterol: 0mg
- Carbohydrates: 7g
- Fiber: 2g

Mexican Antojitos

Prep Time: 20 minutes Cooking Time: 10 minutes Serving Size: 2 antojitos

Ingredients:

- 2 whole wheat tortillas
- 1/2 cup black beans, rinsed and drained
- 1/4 cup red onion, finely chopped
- 1/4 cup tomato, diced
- 1/4 cup bell pepper, diced
- 1/4 teaspoon cumin
- 1/4 teaspoon chili powder
- 1/4 cup low-fat shredded cheddar cheese
- Fresh cilantro, chopped, for garnish
- 1/4 avocado, diced, for garnish

Instructions:

1. Preheat oven to 350°F.

2. In a bowl, mix black beans, red onion, tomato, bell pepper, cumin, and chili powder.

3. Lay out the tortillas and evenly distribute the bean mixture over half of each tortilla. Sprinkle with cheddar cheese.

4. Fold the tortillas in half and press gently to seal.

5. Place on a baking sheet and bake for 10 minutes, until the cheese is melted and the tortillas are slightly crispy.

6. Cut each antojito into 3 pieces, garnish with fresh cilantro and avocado, and serve.

Nutritional Information (per serving):

- Calories: 200
- Protein: 9g
- Sodium: 320mg
- Potassium: 450mg
- Total Fat: 7g
- Saturated Fat: 2g
- Cholesterol: 10mg
- Carbohydrates: 27g
- Fiber: 5g

Moroccan Couscous

Prep Time: 15 minutes Cooking Time: 5
minutes Serving Size: 1 cup

Ingredients:

- 1 cup whole wheat couscous
- 1 1/4 cups low-sodium vegetable broth
- 1/2 teaspoon turmeric
- 1/2 teaspoon cumin
- 1/2 cup carrot, diced
- 1/2 cup zucchini, diced
- 1/4 cup raisins
- 1/4 cup almonds, slivered
- 2 tablespoons fresh parsley, chopped
- 2 tablespoons fresh mint, chopped
- Lemon wedges, for serving

Instructions:

1. In a medium saucepan, bring the vegetable broth to a boil. Add turmeric and cumin.
2. Stir in the couscous, cover, and remove from heat. Let it stand for 5 minutes.
3. Fluff the couscous with a fork. Stir in the carrot, zucchini, raisins, almonds, parsley, and mint.
4. Serve warm or at room temperature with lemon wedges on the side.

Nutritional Information (per serving):

- Calories: 220
- Protein: 7g
- Sodium: 80mg
- Potassium: 300mg
- Total Fat: 4g
- Saturated Fat: 0.5g
- Cholesterol: 0mg
- Carbohydrates: 40g
- Fiber: 6g

Apple Spice Cake

Prep Time: 30 minutes

Cooking Time: 45 minutes

Serving Size: 1 slice

Ingredients:

- 1 1/2 cups all-purpose flour
- 1/2 cup whole wheat flour
- 2 tsp baking powder (aluminum-free)
- 1/2 tsp baking soda
- 1/4 tsp salt
- 2 tsp ground cinnamon
- 1/2 tsp ground nutmeg
- 1/4 cup unsweetened applesauce
- 3/4 cup sugar (or a suitable sugar substitute for a lower calorie option)
- 2 large eggs
- 1/4 cup vegetable oil
- 4 cups peeled and finely chopped apples (about 4 medium apples)
- 1 tsp vanilla extract

Instructions:

1. Preheat the oven to 350°F. Grease and flour a 9-inch round cake pan.
2. In a bowl, whisk together both flours, baking powder, baking soda, salt, cinnamon, and nutmeg.
3. In a separate large bowl, beat together applesauce, sugar, eggs, and oil until smooth.

4. Gradually add the dry ingredients to the wet ingredients, stirring just until combined.

5. Fold in the chopped apples and vanilla extract.

6. Pour the batter into the prepared cake pan and smooth the top with a spatula.

7. Bake for 45 minutes, or until a toothpick inserted into the center comes out clean.

8. Let the cake cool in the pan for 10 minutes, then turn out onto a wire rack to cool completely.

Nutritional Information (per serving):

- Calories: 210
- Protein: 3g
- Sodium: 150mg
- Potassium: 130mg
- Total Fat: 5g
- Saturated Fat: 1g
- Cholesterol: 31mg
- Carbohydrates: 38g
- Fiber: 2g

Roasted Asparagus and Wild Mushroom Stew

Prep Time: 20 minutes

Cooking Time: 30 minutes

Serving Size: 1 cup

Ingredients:

- 1 lb asparagus, trimmed and cut into 2-inch pieces
- 1/2 lb wild mushrooms (e.g., shiitake, oyster), cleaned and sliced
- 2 tbsp olive oil
- 1 medium onion, diced
- 2 cloves garlic, minced
- 4 cups low-sodium vegetable broth
- 1/2 tsp dried thyme
- 1/2 tsp dried rosemary
- 1/4 tsp black pepper
- 1/4 cup low-fat milk or a dairy-free alternative
- 2 tbsp cornstarch mixed with 2 tbsp water

Instructions:

1. Preheat the oven to 425°F. Toss asparagus and mushrooms with 1 tablespoon of olive oil and spread them on a baking sheet. Roast for 20 minutes, or until tender and lightly browned.

2. Meanwhile, in a large pot, heat the remaining olive oil over medium heat. Add the onion and garlic, cooking until soft and translucent.

3. Add the roasted vegetables to the pot along with the vegetable broth, thyme, rosemary, and black pepper. Bring to a simmer.

4. Mix the milk and cornstarch mixture until smooth, then stir into the stew. Continue to cook, stirring frequently, until the stew thickens slightly, about 10 minutes.

5. Adjust seasoning if necessary and serve hot.

Nutritional Information (per serving):

- Calories: 100
- Protein: 3g
- Sodium: 70mg
- Potassium: 300mg
- Total Fat: 5g
- Saturated Fat: 1g
- Cholesterol: 0mg
- Carbohydrates: 12g
- Fiber: 3g

Balsamic Marinated Mushrooms

Prep Time: 15 minutes + Marinating Time

Cooking Time: 0 minutes

Serving Size: 1/4 cup

Ingredients:

- 1 lb fresh button mushrooms, cleaned and halved
- 1/4 cup balsamic vinegar
- 2 tbsp olive oil
- 1 clove garlic, minced
- 1 tsp dried oregano
- 1/4 tsp black pepper
- 2 tbsp fresh parsley, chopped

Instructions:

1. In a large bowl, whisk together balsamic vinegar, olive oil, garlic, oregano, and black pepper.
2. Add the mushrooms to the bowl and toss to coat evenly. Cover and refrigerate for at least 2 hours, or overnight for best flavor, stirring occasionally.
3. Before serving, sprinkle with fresh parsley. Serve chilled or at room temperature.

Nutritional Information (per serving):

- Calories: 50
- Protein: 2g
- Sodium: 10mg
- Potassium: 300mg
- Total Fat: 4g
- Saturated Fat: 0.5g
- Cholesterol: 0mg
- Carbohydrates: 3g
- Fiber: 1g

Blueberry Lemon Pound Cake

Prep Time: 20 minutes

Cooking Time: 60 minutes

Serving Size: 1 slice

Ingredients:

- 1 3/4 cups all-purpose flour
- 1/2 cup whole wheat flour
- 1 tsp baking powder (aluminum-free)
- 1/4 tsp salt
- 1 cup unsweetened applesauce
- 3/4 cup sugar (or a suitable sugar substitute)
- 3 large eggs
- 1/4 cup olive oil
- 1 tsp vanilla extract
- 1 tbsp lemon zest
- 1/4 cup lemon juice
- 1 1/2 cups fresh or frozen (thawed) blueberries

1. Preheat the oven to 350°F. Grease and flour a 9x5-inch loaf pan.
2. In a bowl, whisk together both flours, baking powder, and salt.
3. In a separate large bowl, beat together applesauce, sugar, eggs, olive oil, vanilla extract, lemon zest, and lemon juice until smooth.
4. Gradually add the dry ingredients to the wet ingredients, stirring just until combined.
5. Gently fold in the blueberries.
6. Pour the batter into the prepared loaf pan and smooth the top with a spatula.
7. Bake for 60 minutes, or until a toothpick inserted into the center comes out clean.
8. Let the cake cool in the pan for 10 minutes, then turn out onto a wire rack to cool completely.

Nutritional Information (per serving):

- Calories: 210
- Protein: 4g
- Sodium: 85mg
- Potassium: 115mg
- Total Fat: 6g
- Saturated Fat: 1g
- Cholesterol: 46mg
- Carbohydrates: 34g
- Fiber: 2g

Creamy Curry Rice & Apple Salad

Prep Time: 25 minutes

Cooking Time: 35 minutes

Serving Size: 1 cup

Ingredients:

- 1 cup brown rice, rinsed
- 2 1/4 cups water
- 1/4 teaspoon salt (optional, consider your dietary restrictions)
- 1 tablespoon olive oil
- 1 medium onion, finely chopped
- 1/2 cup celery, chopped
- 1 apple, cored and chopped (choose a sweet variety like Fuji or Gala)
- 1/4 cup raisins
- 1/4 teaspoon ground turmeric
- 1/2 teaspoon curry powder (adjust based on tolerance for spices)
- 1/2 cup unsweetened almond milk
- 2 tablespoons low-fat mayonnaise
- Fresh cilantro for garnish (optional)

Instructions:

1. In a medium saucepan, combine rice, water, and salt. Bring to a boil, then reduce heat to low, cover, and simmer for about 30 minutes, or until rice is tender and water is absorbed. Let it cool.
2. In a skillet, heat olive oil over medium heat. Add onion and celery, and sauté until soft, about 5 minutes.

3. In a large bowl, combine the cooked rice, sautéed onion and celery, chopped apple, and raisins.

4. In a small bowl, mix together turmeric, curry powder, almond milk, and mayonnaise until smooth. Pour over the rice mixture and gently stir to combine.

5. Garnish with fresh cilantro if desired. Serve chilled or at room temperature.

Nutritional Information (per serving):

- Calories: 200
- Protein: 4g
- Sodium: 75mg (without added salt)
- Potassium: 250mg
- Total Fat: 5g
- Saturated Fat: 0.5g
- Cholesterol: 2mg
- Carbohydrates: 36g
- Fiber: 4g

Favorite Cranberry Salad

Prep Time: 15 minutes

Cooking Time: 0 minutes (requires chilling)

Serving Size: 1/2 cup

Ingredients:

- 1 cup fresh cranberries, finely chopped
- 1/2 cup crushed pineapple, drained (canned in juice, not syrup)
- 1/4 cup sugar substitute (e.g., stevia or erythritol blend suitable for cooking)
- 1/2 cup celery, finely chopped
- 1/4 cup walnuts, chopped (optional, depending on dietary restrictions)
- 1 cup unsweetened whipped cream

Instructions:

1. In a bowl, mix together the chopped cranberries and sugar substitute. Let sit for 10 minutes to allow cranberries to soften and become slightly sweetened.

2. Add the drained crushed pineapple and chopped celery to the cranberry mixture.

3. Gently fold in the whipped cream until well combined.

4. If using walnuts, sprinkle them on top or mix them in, depending on preference.

5. Refrigerate for at least an hour before serving to allow flavors to meld.

Nutritional Information (per serving):

- Calories: 90
- Protein: 1g
- Sodium: 20mg
- Potassium: 90mg
- Total Fat: 7g (less if not adding walnuts)
- Saturated Fat: 4g
- Cholesterol: 20mg
- Carbohydrates: 8g
- Fiber: 2g

Gelatin Beet Salad

Prep Time: 15 minutes (plus chilling)

Cooking Time: 0 minutes

Serving Size: 1/2 cup

Ingredients:

- 1 1/2 cups water
- 1 packet unsweetened gelatin powder (about 2 1/2 teaspoons)
- 1/4 cup lemon juice
- 1 tablespoon apple cider vinegar
- 1 tablespoon sugar substitute (e.g., stevia or erythritol blend suitable for cooking)
- 1 cup cooked beets, diced (fresh or canned without added salt or sugar)
- 1/2 cup cucumber, peeled and finely diced
- 1/4 cup red onion, finely chopped

Instructions:

1. In a small saucepan, bring 1/2 cup of water to a boil. Remove from heat and dissolve the gelatin powder in the hot water, stirring until fully dissolved.
2. Add the remaining 1 cup of cold water, lemon juice, apple cider vinegar, and sugar substitute to the gelatin mixture. Stir well.
3. In a mold or deep dish, layer the diced beets, cucumber, and red onion.
4. Pour the gelatin mixture over the vegetables in the mold. Refrigerate until set, at least 4 hours or overnight.
5. To serve, invert the mold onto a plate. If the salad does not release easily, briefly dip the bottom of the mold in warm water.

Nutritional Information (per serving):

- Calories: 30
- Protein: 2g
- Sodium: 30mg
- Potassium: 100mg
- Total Fat: 0g
- Saturated Fat: 0g
- Cholesterol: 0mg
- Carbohydrates: 6g
- Fiber: 1g

Healthy Chicken Nuggets

Prep Time: 15 minutes

Cooking Time: 20 minutes

Serving Size: 4 nuggets

Ingredients:

- 1 pound boneless, skinless chicken breasts, cut into nugget-sized pieces
- 1/4 cup almond flour
- 1/4 cup ground flaxseed
- 1 teaspoon garlic powder
- 1 teaspoon onion powder
- 1/2 teaspoon paprika
- 1/4 teaspoon black pepper
- 1 egg, beaten
- 2 tablespoons olive oil for baking sheet

Instructions:

1. Preheat oven to 375°F (190°C). Lightly grease a baking sheet with olive oil.

2. In a shallow dish, combine almond flour, ground flaxseed, garlic powder, onion powder, paprika, and black pepper.

3. Dip each chicken piece into the beaten egg, then roll in the flour mixture to coat. Place on the prepared baking sheet.

4. Bake for 20 minutes or until chicken is cooked through and the coating is golden.

5. Serve warm with a side of low-sodium dipping sauce or fresh lemon wedges.

Nutritional Information (per serving):

- Calories: 220
- Protein: 26g
- Sodium: 70mg
- Potassium: 250mg
- Total Fat: 11g
- Saturated Fat: 1.5g
- Cholesterol: 85mg
- Carbohydrates: 3g
- Fiber: 2g

Grilled Vegetables with Herbed Vinaigrette

Prep Time: 15 minutes
Cooking Time: 20 minutes
Serving Size: 2 cups of vegetables
Ingredients:

- 2 bell peppers, any color, sliced into large pieces
- 1 large zucchini, sliced lengthwise
- 1 large yellow squash, sliced lengthwise
- 1 medium eggplant, sliced into rounds
- 1 medium red onion, sliced into rounds
- 2 tbsp olive oil
- Fresh ground pepper, to taste

For the Herbed Vinaigrette:

- 3 tbsp olive oil
- 1 tbsp white wine vinegar
- 1 tsp Dijon mustard
- 1 garlic clove, minced
- 1 tbsp fresh parsley, finely chopped
- 1 tbsp fresh basil, finely chopped
- Fresh ground pepper, to taste

Instructions:

1. Preheat the grill to medium-high heat. Gently toss the sliced vegetables in olive oil and season with fresh ground pepper.

2. Place the vegetables on the grill, cooking each side for 3-4 minutes until they have nice grill marks and are tender. Remove from grill and let cool slightly.

3. For the vinaigrette, whisk together olive oil, white wine vinegar, Dijon mustard, minced garlic, parsley, basil, and pepper in a small bowl until well combined.

4. Arrange the grilled vegetables on a serving platter and drizzle with the herbed vinaigrette. Serve either warm or at room temperature.

Nutritional Information (per serving):

- Calories: 180
- Protein: 2g
- Sodium: 45mg
- Potassium: 450mg
- Total Fat: 14g

- Saturated Fat: 2g
- Cholesterol: 0mg
- Carbohydrates: 14g
- Fiber: 5g

Mexican Antojitos

Prep Time: 25 minutes

Cooking Time: 5 minutes

Serving Size: 2 antojitos

Ingredients:

- 4 small corn tortillas
- 1/2 cup low-sodium refried beans
- 1/4 cup red bell pepper, finely diced
- 1/4 cup green bell pepper, finely diced
- 1/4 cup reduced-fat shredded cheese
- 1/2 avocado, diced
- 1/4 cup fresh cilantro, chopped
- 1 lime, cut into wedges

Instructions:

1. Spread each corn tortilla with a layer of low-sodium refried beans. Top with diced red and green bell peppers and a sprinkle of reduced-fat shredded cheese.
2. Warm a non-stick skillet over medium heat. Place the tortillas in the skillet, cooking for 2-3 minutes on each side until the cheese is melted and the tortillas are slightly crispy.
3. Remove from heat, and top each antojito with diced avocado and chopped cilantro. Serve with lime wedges to squeeze over the top.

Nutritional Information (per serving):

- Calories: 250
- Protein: 8g
- Sodium: 150mg
- Potassium: 350mg
- Total Fat: 11g
- Saturated Fat: 3g
- Cholesterol: 15mg
- Carbohydrates: 34g
- Fiber: 8g

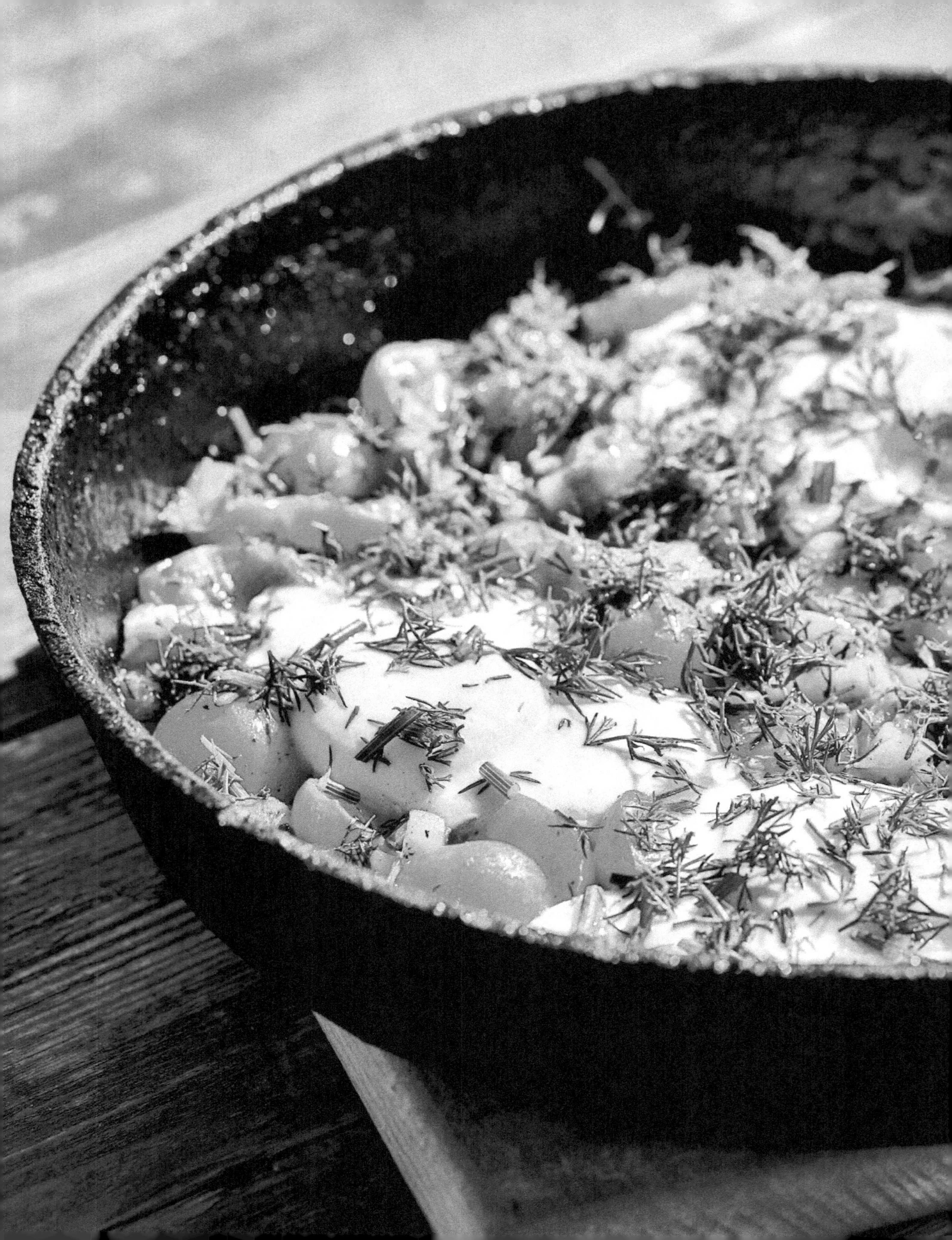

DESSERT

Baked Shrimp Rolls

Prep Time: 25 minutes

Cooking Time: 10 minutes

Serving Size: 2 rolls

Ingredients:

- 12 oz shrimp, peeled and deveined
- 1 tbsp olive oil
- 1/4 cup celery, finely chopped
- 1/4 cup red bell pepper, finely chopped
- 2 tbsp low-fat mayonnaise
- 1 tsp Dijon mustard
- 1 tbsp lemon juice
- 1/2 tsp black pepper
- 4 whole wheat rolls
- 1 cup spinach leaves

Instructions:

1. Preheat oven to 375°F. Toss shrimp with olive oil, spread on a baking sheet, and bake for 8-10 minutes until pink and cooked through.
2. Chop cooked shrimp and mix with celery, red bell pepper, mayonnaise, Dijon mustard, lemon juice, and black pepper.
3. Cut the top off each roll and hollow out the insides. Fill each roll with the shrimp mixture and top with spinach leaves.
4. Serve immediately or wrap in foil to keep warm until serving.

Nutritional Information (per serving):

- Calories: 290
- Protein: 24g
- Sodium: 410mg
- Potassium: 330mg
- Total Fat: 8g
- Saturated Fat: 1g
- Cholesterol: 182mg
- Carbohydrates: 29g
- Fiber: 5g

Barbecue Meatballs

Prep Time: 20 minutes

Cooking Time: 25 minutes

Serving Size: 4 meatballs

Ingredients:

- 1 lb ground turkey breast
- 1/4 cup whole wheat breadcrumbs
- 1 egg white
- 1/4 cup onion, finely chopped
- 1/2 tsp garlic powder
- 1/2 cup low-sodium barbecue sauce
- 1/4 cup water

Instructions:

1. Preheat oven to 375°F. Combine ground turkey, breadcrumbs, egg white, onion, and garlic powder in a bowl.
2. Form into 16 meatballs and place on a baking sheet lined with parchment paper.

3. Bake for 15 minutes. In a saucepan, mix barbecue sauce and water, and bring to a simmer.

4. Add baked meatballs to the saucepan, cover, and simmer for an additional 10 minutes.

5. Serve hot.

Nutritional Information (per serving):

- Calories: 165
- Protein: 22g
- Sodium: 240mg
- Potassium: 310mg
- Total Fat: 2g
- Saturated Fat: 0.5g
- Cholesterol: 55mg
- Carbohydrates: 15g
- Fiber: 1g

Brie and Cranberry Chutney

Prep Time: 10 minutes

Cooking Time: 20 minutes

Serving Size: 1 tablespoon chutney with 1 ounce brie

Ingredients:

- 1 cup fresh cranberries
- 1/4 cup orange juice
- 2 tbsp honey
- 1/4 tsp ground cinnamon
- 1/4 tsp ground ginger
- 8 oz brie cheese, cut into 1 oz servings

Instructions:

1. Combine cranberries, orange juice, honey, cinnamon, and ginger in a saucepan over medium heat.

2. Cook until cranberries have popped and the mixture has thickened, about 20 minutes.

3. Let cool slightly before serving over brie cheese slices.

Nutritional Information (per serving):

- Calories: 100
- Protein: 6g
- Sodium: 180mg
- Potassium: 60mg
- Total Fat: 7g
- Saturated Fat: 4g
- Cholesterol: 28mg
- Carbohydrates: 5g
- Fiber: 1g

Brown Sugar Apple Dip

Prep Time: 5 minutes

Cooking Time: 0 minutes

Serving Size: 2 tablespoons

Ingredients:

- 1 cup low-fat plain Greek yogurt
- 2 tbsp brown sugar
- 1/2 tsp vanilla extract
- 1/4 tsp ground cinnamon
- Apple slices for serving

Instructions:

1. Mix Greek yogurt, brown sugar, vanilla extract, and cinnamon in a bowl until well combined.
2. Serve immediately with apple slices, or refrigerate until ready to serve.

Nutritional Information (per serving):

- Calories: 45
- Protein: 4g
- Sodium: 25mg
- Potassium: 60mg
- Total Fat: 0.5g
- Saturated Fat: 0g
- Cholesterol: 2mg
- Carbohydrates: 8g
- Fiber: 0g

Buffalo Chicken Dip

Prep Time: 20 minutes

Cooking Time: 25 minutes

Serving Size: ¼ cup

Ingredients:

- 1 lb chicken breast, cooked and shredded
- 8 oz low-fat cream cheese, softened
- ½ cup low-sodium Greek yogurt
- ¼ cup hot sauce (check sodium content, choose low-sodium)
- 1 tsp garlic powder
- 1 tsp onion powder
- ½ cup shredded low-fat cheddar cheese
- 2 tbsp fresh chives, chopped

Instructions:

1. Preheat your oven to 350°F. In a mixing bowl, combine the cooked shredded chicken, softened cream cheese, Greek yogurt, and hot sauce until the mixture is uniform.
2. Stir in the garlic powder and onion powder, ensuring they're well distributed throughout the mix.
3. Transfer the chicken mixture to a baking dish, spreading it evenly. Sprinkle the shredded cheddar cheese over the top.
4. Bake in the preheated oven for 20-25 minutes, or until the cheese is bubbly and slightly golden.
5. Garnish with chopped chives before serving. Enjoy with fresh vegetable sticks or low-sodium crackers.

Nutritional Information (per serving):

- Calories: 135
- Protein: 14g
- Sodium: 180mg
- Potassium: 190mg
- Total Fat: 6g
- Saturated Fat: 3g
- Cholesterol: 40mg
- Carbohydrates: 3g
- Fiber: 0g

Buffalo Wings

Prep Time: 15 minutes

Cooking Time: 45 minutes

Serving Size: 2 wings

Ingredients:

- 2 lbs chicken wings, skin removed
- 1 tbsp olive oil
- 1 tsp garlic powder
- 1 tsp paprika
- ¼ cup low-sodium hot sauce
- 1 tbsp vinegar
- 1 tbsp honey
- Fresh ground pepper, to taste

Instructions:

1. Preheat your oven to 400°F. Toss the skinless chicken wings with olive oil, garlic powder, and paprika.
2. Arrange the wings on a baking sheet lined with parchment paper, ensuring they're not touching.
3. Bake for 45 minutes, flipping halfway through, until they are crispy and fully cooked.
4. While the wings are baking, whisk together the low-sodium hot sauce, vinegar, and honey in a bowl.
5. Once the wings are done, toss them in the sauce mixture until they're well coated. Serve immediately, garnished with fresh ground pepper.

Nutritional Information (per serving):

- Calories: 210
- Protein: 22g
- Sodium: 200mg
- Potassium: 220mg
- Total Fat: 10g
- Saturated Fat: 2.5g
- Cholesterol: 80mg
- Carbohydrates: 5g
- Fiber: 0.5g

Cereal Snack Mix with Salt-free Seasoning

Prep Time: 10 minutes

Cooking Time: 0 minutes

Serving Size: ½ cup

Ingredients:

- 2 cups puffed rice cereal
- 1 cup whole grain oats
- ½ cup unsalted almonds, chopped
- ¼ cup pumpkin seeds
- 2 tbsp dried cranberries
- 1 tsp dried rosemary, crushed
- 1 tsp dried thyme
- 1 tsp garlic powder
- ½ tsp onion powder
- ¼ tsp black pepper

Instructions:

1. In a large bowl, mix together the puffed rice cereal, whole grain oats, chopped almonds, pumpkin seeds, and dried cranberries.
2. Add the dried rosemary, thyme, garlic powder, onion powder, and black pepper to the mix. Stir until all the ingredients are evenly seasoned.

3. Store the snack mix in an airtight container. It can be enjoyed immediately or saved for later as a kidney-friendly, heart-healthy snack.

Nutritional Information (per serving):

- Calories: 120
- Protein: 4g
- Sodium: 15mg
- Potassium: 150mg
- Total Fat: 5g
- Saturated Fat: 0.5g
- Cholesterol: 0mg
- Carbohydrates: 16g
- Fiber: 3g

Chicken Nuggets with Honey Mustard Dipping Sauce

Prep Time: 15 minutes

Cooking Time: 20 minutes

Serving Size: 4 nuggets

Ingredients:

For the Nuggets:

- 1 lb chicken breast, cut into nugget-sized pieces
- ½ cup almond flour
- 1 egg, beaten
- 1 tsp garlic powder
- 1 tsp paprika
- Olive oil spray

For the Dipping Sauce:

- ¼ cup low-fat Greek yogurt
- 1 tbsp honey
- 1 tbsp mustard (check for low-sodium options)
- 1 tsp lemon juice

Instructions:

1. Preheat your oven to 400°F. Line a baking sheet with parchment paper.
2. In a shallow dish, combine the almond flour, garlic powder, and paprika.
3. Dip each chicken piece into the beaten egg, then coat with the almond flour mixture.
4. Arrange the coated chicken pieces on the prepared baking sheet and lightly spray with olive oil.
5. Bake for 20 minutes, flipping halfway through, until the nuggets are golden and cooked through.
6. While the nuggets are baking, prepare the dipping sauce by mixing together the Greek yogurt, honey, mustard, and lemon juice in a small bowl.
7. Serve the chicken nuggets hot with the honey mustard dipping sauce on the side.

Nutritional Information (per serving):

- Calories: 220
- Protein: 26g
- Sodium: 150mg
- Potassium: 300mg
- Total Fat: 9g
- Saturated Fat: 1.5g
- Cholesterol: 90mg
- Carbohydrates: 8g
- Fiber: 2g

Chicken Parmesan Meatballs

Prep Time: 30 minutes

Cooking Time: 20 minutes

Serving Size: 2 meatballs

Ingredients:

- 1 lb ground chicken breast
- 1/4 cup almond flour
- 1 large egg
- 1/2 cup grated Parmesan cheese
- 2 tbsp chopped fresh basil
- 1 tsp garlic powder
- 1/2 tsp onion powder
- 1/4 tsp black pepper
- 2 cups homemade low-sodium tomato sauce
- 1/2 cup shredded mozzarella cheese (low-fat)
- Cooking spray

Instructions:

1. Preheat the oven to 375°F. Lightly grease a baking sheet with cooking spray.
2. In a large bowl, combine ground chicken, almond flour, egg, Parmesan cheese, basil, garlic powder, onion powder, and black pepper. Mix well until all ingredients are evenly distributed.
3. Form the mixture into meatballs, about the size of a golf ball, and place them on the prepared baking sheet.
4. Bake in the preheated oven for 15 minutes, or until the meatballs are cooked through.
5. Heat the tomato sauce in a large pan over medium heat. Add the baked meatballs to the sauce, coating them well. Simmer for 5 minutes.
6. Sprinkle mozzarella cheese over the meatballs and sauce. Cover the pan and cook for an additional 5 minutes, or until the cheese is melted and bubbly.
7. Serve hot, garnished with extra basil if desired.

Nutritional Information (per serving):

- Calories: 220
- Protein: 28g
- Sodium: 290mg
- Potassium: 450mg
- Total Fat: 9g
- Saturated Fat: 3g
- Cholesterol: 98mg
- Carbohydrates: 8g
- Fiber: 2g

Chicken Pepper Bacon Wraps

Prep Time: 20 minutes

Cooking Time: 25 minutes

Serving Size: 2 wraps

Ingredients:

- 1 lb chicken breast, thinly sliced
- 1 tsp olive oil
- 1/4 tsp black pepper
- 1/2 tsp smoked paprika
- 1 bell pepper, sliced
- 8 slices of turkey bacon
- 1 tbsp low-sodium soy sauce

Instructions:

1. Preheat the oven to 400°F.
2. Toss the chicken slices with olive oil, black pepper, and smoked paprika.
3. Wrap each chicken slice with a slice of bell pepper and then with turkey bacon, securing with a toothpick if necessary.
4. Arrange the wraps on a baking sheet and lightly brush each with low-sodium soy sauce.
5. Bake for 25 minutes, or until the bacon is crisp and the chicken is cooked through.
6. Serve immediately, with extra soy sauce for dipping if desired.

Nutritional Information (per serving):

- Calories: 265
- Protein: 38g
- Sodium: 585mg
- Potassium: 650mg
- Total Fat: 8g
- Saturated Fat: 2g
- Cholesterol: 95mg
- Carbohydrates: 5g
- Fiber: 1g

Crispy-Crunch Snack Bars

Prep Time: 15 minutes

Cooking Time: 0 minutes (Refrigerate for 2 hours)

Serving Size: 1 bar

Ingredients:

- 1 cup puffed quinoa
- 1/2 cup unsalted nuts (almonds, walnuts), chopped
- 1/4 cup pumpkin seeds
- 1/4 cup unsweetened shredded coconut
- 1/4 cup dried cranberries, no added sugar
- 1/2 cup almond butter
- 1/4 cup honey
- 1 tsp vanilla extract

Instructions:

1. Line a baking pan with parchment paper.
2. In a large bowl, mix together puffed quinoa, chopped nuts, pumpkin seeds, shredded coconut, and dried cranberries.
3. In a small saucepan over low heat, melt almond butter with honey and vanilla extract, stirring until smooth.
4. Pour the almond butter mixture over the dry ingredients and stir until well coated.
5. Spread the mixture evenly in the prepared baking pan, pressing down firmly.
6. Refrigerate for at least 2 hours, or until set. Cut into bars.
7. Store in an airtight container in the refrigerator.

Nutritional Information (per serving):

- Calories: 150
- Protein: 4g
- Sodium: 10mg
- Potassium: 135mg
- Total Fat: 9g
- Saturated Fat: 1g
- Cholesterol: 0mg
- Carbohydrates: 15g
- Fiber: 2g

Falafel

Prep Time: 15 minutes (plus soaking time for chickpeas)

Cooking Time: 10 minutes

Serving Size: 4 falafels

Ingredients:

- 1 cup dried chickpeas, soaked overnight and drained
- 1/4 cup onion, chopped
- 2 cloves garlic
- 1/4 cup fresh parsley, chopped
- 1 tsp ground cumin
- 1 tsp ground coriander
- 1/4 tsp black pepper
- 1/4 tsp cayenne pepper (optional)
- 1 tsp lemon juice
- 1/2 tsp baking soda
- 2 tbsp whole wheat flour
- Olive oil spray for cooking

Instructions:

1. In a food processor, combine soaked chickpeas, onion, garlic, parsley, cumin, coriander, black pepper, cayenne pepper (if using), and lemon juice. Process until mixture is smooth.

2. Transfer to a bowl and stir in baking soda and whole wheat flour. Let the mixture rest for 10 minutes.

3. Form the mixture into small balls or patties.

4. Heat a non-stick pan over medium heat and lightly spray with olive oil. Cook the falafel in batches, turning occasionally, until golden and crispy, about 5 minutes on each side.

5. Serve hot with a side of low-sodium, homemade tzatziki sauce or on a bed of mixed greens.

Nutritional Information (per serving):

- Calories: 198
- Protein: 9g
- Sodium: 175mg
- Potassium: 409mg
- Total Fat: 4g
- Saturated Fat: 0.5g
- Cholesterol: 0mg
- Carbohydrates: 33g
- Fiber: 9g

Flour Tortilla Chips

Prep Time: 10 minutes

Cooking Time: 15 minutes

Serving Size: 6 chips

Ingredients:

- 4 medium whole wheat tortillas (look for low sodium versions)
- 1 tablespoon olive oil
- A pinch of garlic powder
- A pinch of ground black pepper
- A pinch of dried oregano

Instructions:

1. Preheat your oven to 350°F (175°C). Lightly brush each tortilla on one side with olive oil. Stack the tortillas, oiled side up, and cut into sixths to create chips.
2. Spread the tortilla wedges in a single layer on a baking sheet. Sprinkle lightly with garlic powder, black pepper, and dried oregano for flavor.
3. Bake in the preheated oven until the chips are crispy and golden brown, about 12 to 15 minutes. Rotate the baking sheet halfway through for even baking.
4. Allow the chips to cool on the baking sheet for a few minutes before serving. This will help them crisp up further.

Nutritional Information (per serving):

- Calories: 60
- Protein: 2g
- Sodium: 50mg
- Potassium: 30mg
- Total Fat: 2.5g
- Saturated Fat: 0.3g
- Cholesterol: 0mg
- Carbohydrates: 9g
- Fiber: 1g

Garlic Oyster Crackers

Prep Time: 5 minutes

Cooking Time: 15 minutes

Serving Size: 1/2 cup

Ingredients:

- 2 cups oyster crackers (preferably low sodium)
- 1 tablespoon olive oil
- 1/2 teaspoon garlic powder
- 1/4 teaspoon dried parsley
- A pinch of ground black pepper

Instructions:

1. Preheat your oven to 350°F (175°C). In a large bowl, toss the oyster crackers with olive oil, garlic powder, dried parsley, and black pepper until evenly coated.
2. Spread the crackers in a single layer on a baking sheet.
3. Bake for 15 minutes, stirring once at the halfway mark to ensure even toasting.
4. Remove from oven and let cool on the baking sheet. The crackers will become crisper as they cool.

Nutritional Information (per serving):

- Calories: 70
- Protein: 1g

- Sodium: 60mg
- Potassium: 20mg
- Total Fat: 3.5g
- Saturated Fat: 0.5g
- Cholesterol: 0mg
- Carbohydrates: 9g
- Fiber: 0g

Lemon Pepper Hummus

Prep Time: 15 minutes

Cooking Time: 0 minutes

Serving Size: 2 tablespoons

Ingredients:

- 1 can (15 ounces) low-sodium chickpeas, drained and rinsed
- 2 tablespoons fresh lemon juice
- 1 clove garlic, minced
- 1/2 teaspoon ground black pepper
- 1 tablespoon olive oil
- 1/4 teaspoon lemon zest

Instructions:

1. Combine chickpeas, lemon juice, garlic, and black pepper in a food processor. Blend until smooth.
2. While blending, slowly add olive oil until the mixture is creamy.
3. Stir in lemon zest for added flavor.
4. Serve chilled or at room temperature.

Nutritional Information (per serving):

- Calories: 68
- Protein: 2g
- Sodium: 80mg
- Potassium: 84mg

- Total Fat: 3g
- Saturated Fat: 0.4g
- Cholesterol: 0mg
- Carbohydrates: 8g
- Fiber: 2g

Pickled Okra

Prep Time: 25 minutes

Cooking Time: 5 minutes

Serving Size: 1 okra

Ingredients:

- 1 pound fresh okra
- 2 cups water
- 1 cup white vinegar (5% acidity)
- 2 tablespoons sugar substitute (suitable for cooking)
- 1 teaspoon mustard seeds
- 2 cloves garlic, peeled
- 2 fresh dill sprigs

Instructions:

1. Sterilize jars and lids by boiling them in water for 10 minutes.
2. In a large pot, combine water, vinegar, sugar substitute, and mustard seeds. Bring to a boil.
3. Pack okra into jars, adding 1 garlic clove and 1 dill sprig to each jar.
4. Pour the boiling vinegar mixture over the okra, leaving 1/2-inch headspace. Seal jars.
5. Process in a boiling water bath for 10 minutes. Remove and let cool.

6. Check seals and store in a cool, dark place for up to a year.

Nutritional Information (per serving):

- Calories: 8
- Protein: 0.5g
- Sodium: 2mg
- Potassium: 60mg
- Total Fat: 0.1g
- Saturated Fat: 0g
- Cholesterol: 0mg
- Carbohydrates: 1.9g
- Fiber: 0.6g

Raspberry Wings

Prep Time: 10 minutes (plus marinating time)

Cooking Time: 20 minutes

Serving Size: 4 wings

Ingredients:

- 12 chicken wings, skin removed
- 1/2 cup fresh raspberries
- 2 tablespoons balsamic vinegar
- 1 tablespoon olive oil
- 1 teaspoon honey substitute (suitable for cooking)
- 1 clove garlic, minced
- 1/4 teaspoon ground black pepper

Instructions:

1. Puree raspberries, balsamic vinegar, olive oil, honey substitute, garlic, and black pepper in a blender until smooth.
2. Marinate chicken wings in the raspberry mixture for at least 2 hours in the refrigerator, preferably overnight.
3. Preheat oven to 375°F. Place wings on a baking sheet lined with parchment paper.
4. Bake for 20 minutes, or until fully cooked and juices run clear, turning once halfway through.
5. Serve hot.

Nutritional Information (per serving):

- Calories: 190
- Protein: 15g
- Sodium: 70mg
- Potassium: 150mg
- Total Fat: 10g
- Saturated Fat: 2g
- Cholesterol: 42mg
- Carbohydrates: 5g
- Fiber: 1g

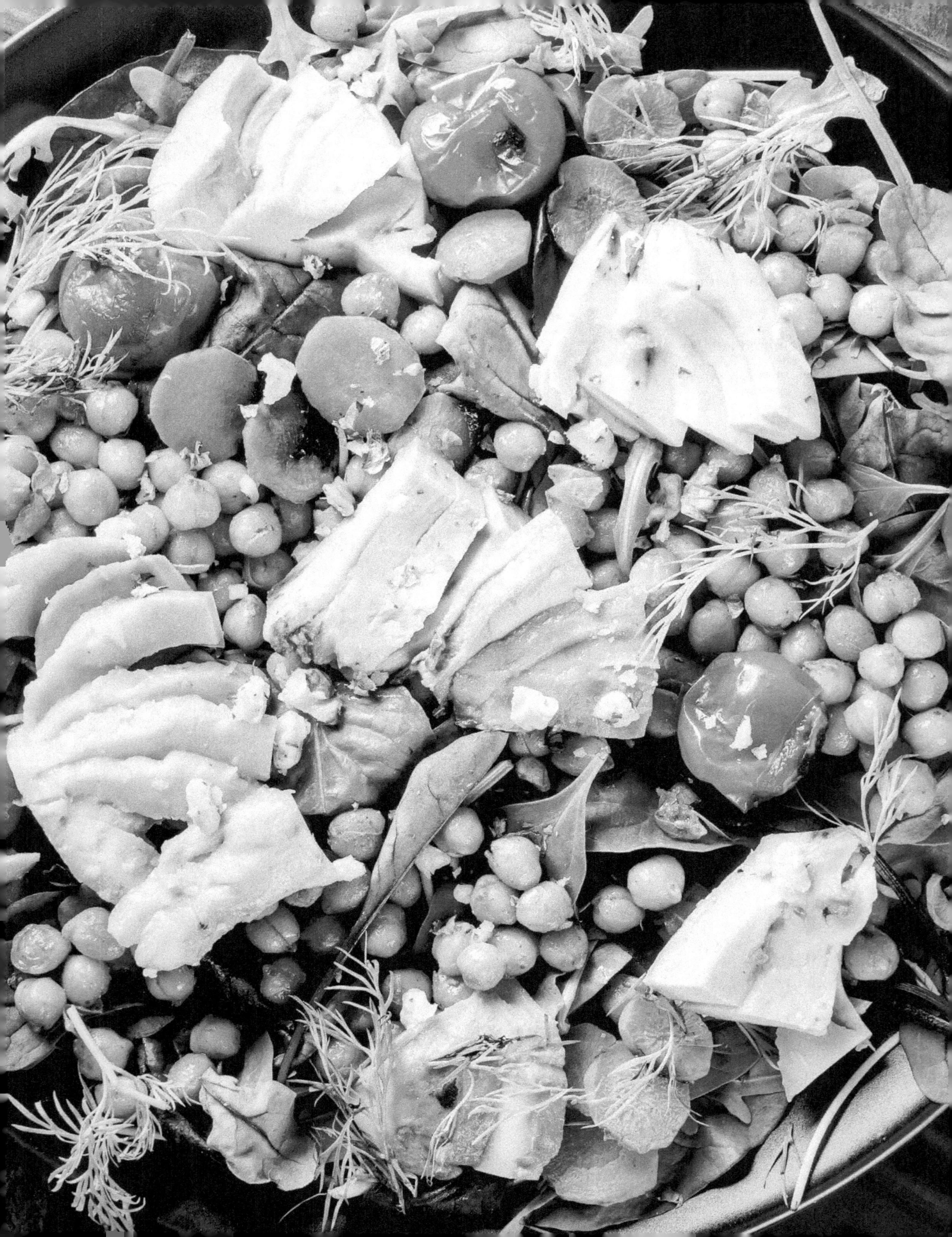

SALADS & SALAD DRESSINGS

Apple Cranberry Slaw with Celery Seed Dressing

Prep Time: 15 minutes

Cooking Time: 0 minutes (chill for at least 1 hour before serving)

Serving Size: 1 cup

Ingredients:

- 2 cups green cabbage, shredded
- 1 apple, preferably a tart variety like Granny Smith, julienne
- 1/4 cup dried cranberries, low sugar
- 2 tablespoons red onion, finely chopped
- 2 tablespoons apple cider vinegar
- 1 tablespoon olive oil
- 1/2 teaspoon celery seed
- 1 teaspoon honey (optional)
- Salt (optional) and pepper to taste

Instructions:

1. In a large mixing bowl, combine the shredded cabbage, julienned apple, dried cranberries, and red onion.
2. In a small bowl, whisk together apple cider vinegar, olive oil, celery seed, and honey if using. Season with a pinch of salt (optional) and pepper to taste.
3. Pour the dressing over the cabbage mixture and toss until everything is well coated.
4. Cover and refrigerate for at least 1 hour to allow the flavors to meld. Serve chilled.

Nutritional Information (per serving):

- Calories: 90
- Protein: 1g
- Sodium: 20mg
- Potassium: 150mg
- Total Fat: 3.5g
- Saturated Fat: 0.5g
- Cholesterol: 0mg
- Carbohydrates: 15g
- Fiber: 2g

Asian Cabbage Slaw

Prep Time: 20 minutes

Cooking Time: 0 minutes (chill for at least 30 minutes before serving)

Serving Size: 1 cup

Ingredients:

- 2 cups red cabbage, shredded
- 1 carrot, julienned
- 1/4 cup cucumber, thinly sliced
- 1 tablespoon rice vinegar
- 1 tablespoon sesame oil
- 1 teaspoon soy sauce, low sodium
- 1/2 teaspoon ginger, grated
- 1/2 teaspoon garlic, minced
- 1 tablespoon sesame seeds, toasted

Instructions:

1. In a large bowl, mix the shredded red cabbage, julienned carrot, and thinly sliced cucumber.

2. In a small bowl, whisk together rice vinegar, sesame oil, low sodium soy sauce, grated ginger, and minced garlic to create the dressing.

3. Pour the dressing over the cabbage mixture and toss to combine thoroughly.

4. Sprinkle toasted sesame seeds over the slaw.

5. Chill in the refrigerator for at least 30 minutes before serving to enhance the flavors.

Nutritional Information (per serving):

- Calories: 70
- Protein: 2g
- Sodium: 80mg
- Potassium: 220mg
- Total Fat: 5g
- Saturated Fat: 0.7g
- Cholesterol: 0mg
- Carbohydrates: 6g
- Fiber: 2g

Basil-Lime Pineapple Fruit Salad

Prep Time: 15 minutes

Cooking Time: 0 minutes

Serving Size: 1 cup

Ingredients:

- 2 cups pineapple, cubed
- 1 banana, sliced
- 1/4 cup strawberries, halved
- 2 tablespoons lime juice
- 1 teaspoon lime zest
- 1 tablespoon fresh basil, chopped
- 1 teaspoon honey (optional)

Instructions:

1. In a large bowl, combine the cubed pineapple, sliced banana, and halved strawberries.

2. In a small bowl, mix together lime juice, lime zest, chopped basil, and honey if using.

3. Drizzle the lime-basil dressing over the fruit and gently toss to combine.

4. Serve immediately or chill in the refrigerator for a refreshing, tangy fruit salad.

Nutritional Information (per serving):

- Calories: 70
- Protein: 1g
- Sodium: 5mg
- Potassium: 180mg
- Total Fat: 0g
- Saturated Fat: 0g
- Cholesterol: 0mg
- Carbohydrates: 18g

- Fiber: 2g

Broccoli and Apple Salad

Prep Time: 20 minutes

Cooking Time: 0 minutes

Serving Size: 1 cup

Ingredients:

- 2 cups broccoli florets, finely chopped
- 1 apple, cored and chopped
- 1/4 cup red onion, finely chopped
- 2 tablespoons dried cranberries, low sugar
- 2 tablespoons walnuts, chopped (optional)
- 2 tablespoons Greek yogurt, low-fat
- 1 tablespoon mayonnaise, low-fat
- 1 tablespoon apple cider vinegar
- 1 teaspoon honey (optional)
- Salt (optional) and pepper to taste

Instructions:

1. In a large bowl, combine broccoli florets, chopped apple, red onion, dried cranberries, and walnuts if using.
2. In a separate small bowl, whisk together Greek yogurt, low-fat mayonnaise, apple cider vinegar, and honey if using. Season with a pinch of salt (optional) and pepper to taste.
3. Pour the dressing over the broccoli mixture and toss until well combined.
4. Serve immediately or chill in the refrigerator before serving for enhanced flavors.

Nutritional Information (per serving):

- Calories: 100
- Protein: 3g
- Sodium: 50mg
- Potassium: 250mg
- Total Fat: 4g
- Saturated Fat: 0.5g
- Cholesterol: 1mg
- Carbohydrates: 15g
- Fiber: 3g

Carrot and Jicama Salad

Prep Time: 15 minutes

Cooking Time: 0 minutes

Serving Size: 1 cup

Ingredients:

- 2 cups carrots, julienned
- 1 cup jicama, julienned
- 1/4 cup red onion, thinly sliced
- 2 tablespoons cilantro, chopped
- 3 tablespoons rice vinegar
- 1 tablespoon olive oil
- 1 teaspoon honey
- 1/4 teaspoon ground black pepper

Instructions:

1. In a large bowl, combine the julienned carrots, jicama, thinly sliced red onion, and chopped cilantro.
2. In a small bowl, whisk together rice vinegar, olive oil, honey, and ground black pepper to create the dressing.

3. Pour the dressing over the salad and toss well to ensure everything is evenly coated.

4. Let the salad sit for about 10 minutes before serving to allow the flavors to meld together.

Nutritional Information (per serving):

- Calories: 70
- Protein: 1g
- Sodium: 45mg
- Potassium: 180mg
- Total Fat: 3.5g
- Saturated Fat: 0.5g
- Cholesterol: 0mg
- Carbohydrates: 10g
- Fiber: 3g

Celery Seed Dressing

Prep Time: 5 minutes
Cooking Time: 0 minutes
Serving Size: 1 tablespoon
Ingredients:

- 1/4 cup apple cider vinegar
- 2 tablespoons olive oil
- 1 tablespoon water
- 1 teaspoon honey
- 1 teaspoon celery seeds
- 1/4 teaspoon garlic powder
- 1/4 teaspoon ground black pepper

Instructions:

1. In a small bowl, whisk together all the ingredients until well combined.

2. Store the dressing in an airtight container in the refrigerator. Shake well before each use.

Nutritional Information (per serving):

- Calories: 35
- Protein: 0g
- Sodium: 2mg
- Potassium: 5mg
- Total Fat: 3.5g
- Saturated Fat: 0.5g
- Cholesterol: 0mg
- Carbohydrates: 1g
- Fiber: 0g

Chicken Apple Crunch Salad

Prep Time: 20 minutes
Cooking Time: 0 minutes
Serving Size: 1 cup
Ingredients:

- 2 cups cooked chicken breast, diced
- 1 medium apple, diced
- 1/4 cup celery, diced
- 1/4 cup red bell pepper, diced
- 2 tablespoons walnuts, chopped (optional)
- 1/4 cup Greek yogurt, unsweetened
- 1 tablespoon lemon juice
- 1/4 teaspoon ground black pepper

Instructions:

1. In a large bowl, combine the diced chicken, apple, celery, red bell pepper, and walnuts (if using).

2. In a small bowl, mix together Greek yogurt, lemon juice, and black pepper to make the dressing.

3. Pour the dressing over the salad and toss until everything is evenly coated.

4. Chill for about 30 minutes before serving to enhance the flavors.

Nutritional Information (per serving):

- Calories: 150
- Protein: 18g
- Sodium: 70mg
- Potassium: 250mg
- Total Fat: 4.5g
- Saturated Fat: 1g
- Cholesterol: 45mg
- Carbohydrates: 9g
- Fiber: 2g

Cranberry Dijon Vinaigrette Dressing

Prep Time: 5 minutes

Cooking Time: 0 minutes

Serving Size: 1 tablespoon

Ingredients:

- 1/4 cup cranberry juice (unsweetened)
- 2 tablespoons red wine vinegar
- 1 tablespoon Dijon mustard
- 1 tablespoon olive oil
- 1 teaspoon honey
- 1/4 teaspoon garlic powder
- 1/4 teaspoon ground black pepper

Instructions:

1. In a small bowl, whisk together cranberry juice, red wine vinegar, Dijon mustard, olive oil, honey, garlic powder, and black pepper until well combined.

2. Store in an airtight container in the refrigerator. Shake well before use.

Nutritional Information (per serving):

- Calories: 25
- Protein: 0g
- Sodium: 55mg
- Potassium: 15mg
- Total Fat: 2.5g
- Saturated Fat: 0.3g
- Cholesterol: 0mg
- Carbohydrates: 1g
- Fiber: 0g

Creamy Cucumber Salad

Prep Time: 15 minutes

Cooking Time: 0 minutes

Serving Size: 1 cup

Ingredients:

- 2 medium cucumbers, thinly sliced
- 1/4 cup red onion, thinly sliced
- 1/4 cup Greek yogurt, unsweetened
- 1 tablespoon lemon juice
- 1 teaspoon dill, fresh or dried
- 1/4 teaspoon garlic powder
- 1/4 teaspoon ground black pepper

Instructions:

1. In a large bowl, combine the thinly sliced cucumbers and red onion.

2. In a small bowl, mix together Greek yogurt, lemon juice, dill, garlic powder, and black pepper to make the dressing.

3. Pour the dressing over the cucumber and onion, tossing well to coat.

4. Refrigerate for at least 30 minutes before serving to allow the flavors to develop.

Nutritional Information (per serving):

- Calories: 45
- Protein: 2g
- Sodium: 10mg
- Potassium: 200mg
- Total Fat: 0.5g
- Saturated Fat: 0g
- Cholesterol: 0mg
- Carbohydrates: 8g
- Fiber: 1g

Creamy Fruit Salad

Prep Time: 15 minutes

Serving Size: 1/2 cup

Ingredients:

- 1 cup pineapple chunks, fresh or canned in juice (drained)
- 1 cup strawberries, sliced
- 1 banana, sliced
- 1/2 cup seedless grapes, halved
- 1/4 cup unsweetened shredded coconut
- 1/2 cup Greek yogurt, plain, non-fat
- 1 tbsp honey
- 1 tsp vanilla extract

Instructions:

1. In a large bowl, combine the pineapple, strawberries, banana, and grapes.

2. In a separate small bowl, mix the Greek yogurt, honey, and vanilla extract until well blended.

3. Pour the yogurt dressing over the fruit and gently mix to coat all the fruit pieces evenly. Sprinkle with shredded coconut before serving.

Nutritional Information (per serving):

- Calories: 95
- Protein: 2g
- Sodium: 20mg
- Potassium: 200mg
- Total Fat: 1g
- Saturated Fat: 0.5g
- Cholesterol: 0mg
- Carbohydrates: 20g
- Fiber: 2g

Green Pepper Slaw

Prep Time: 20 minutes

Serving Size: 1/2 cup

Ingredients:

- 2 cups green cabbage, thinly sliced
- 1 green bell pepper, thinly sliced
- 1 carrot, shredded
- 2 tbsp apple cider vinegar
- 1 tbsp olive oil
- 1 tsp honey
- 1/4 tsp black pepper
- 1 tbsp fresh parsley, chopped

Instructions:

1. In a large bowl, combine cabbage, green bell pepper, and carrot.

2. In a small bowl, whisk together apple cider vinegar, olive oil, honey, and black pepper.

3. Pour the dressing over the slaw and toss to combine. Sprinkle with fresh parsley before serving.

Nutritional Information (per serving):

- Calories: 45
- Protein: 1g
- Sodium: 25mg
- Potassium: 150mg
- Total Fat: 2.5g
- Saturated Fat: 0g
- Cholesterol: 0mg
- Carbohydrates: 5g
- Fiber: 2g

Grilled Chicken Salad

Prep Time: 20 minutes

Cooking Time: 10 minutes

Serving Size: 1 cup

Ingredients:

- 4 oz chicken breast, boneless, skinless
- 2 cups mixed greens
- 1/4 cup cucumber, sliced
- 1/4 cup red bell pepper, sliced
- 1 tbsp olive oil
- 2 tbsp balsamic vinegar
- 1/4 tsp garlic powder
- 1/4 tsp black pepper
- 1 tbsp almonds, slivered

Instructions:

1. Season chicken breast with garlic powder and black pepper. Grill over medium heat until fully cooked, about 5 minutes per side. Let it cool and then slice thinly.

2. In a large bowl, combine mixed greens, cucumber, and red bell pepper.

3. Top the salad with sliced chicken and slivered almonds.

4. Drizzle with olive oil and balsamic vinegar before serving.

Nutritional Information (per serving):

- Calories: 225
- Protein: 26g
- Sodium: 65mg
- Potassium: 400mg
- Total Fat: 9g
- Saturated Fat: 1g
- Cholesterol: 65mg
- Carbohydrates: 8g
- Fiber: 2g

Lettuce and Mushroom Salad

Prep Time: 15 minutes

Serving Size: 1 cup

Ingredients:

- 2 cups butter lettuce, torn into pieces
- 1 cup mushrooms, thinly sliced
- 1/4 cup red onion, thinly sliced
- 2 tbsp white wine vinegar
- 1 tbsp olive oil
- 1/2 tsp mustard, Dijon
- 1/4 tsp black pepper
- 1 tbsp chives, chopped

Instructions:

1. In a large salad bowl, combine the butter lettuce, mushrooms, and red onion.

2. In a small bowl, whisk together white wine vinegar, olive oil, Dijon mustard, and black pepper to create the dressing.

3. Pour the dressing over the salad and gently toss to combine. Sprinkle with chopped chives before serving.

Nutritional Information (per serving):

- Calories: 60
- Protein: 2g
- Sodium: 30mg
- Potassium: 250mg
- Total Fat: 5g
- Saturated Fat: 0.7g
- Cholesterol: 0mg
- Carbohydrates: 4g
- Fiber: 1g

Lime Caribbean Dressing

Prep Time: 5 minutes

Serving Size: 2 tablespoons

Ingredients:

- 1/4 cup lime juice, fresh
- 1/4 cup olive oil
- 1 tsp honey
- 1/2 tsp garlic, minced
- 1/4 tsp ground cumin
- 1/8 tsp black pepper
- 1 tbsp cilantro, finely chopped

Instructions:

1. In a small bowl, whisk together lime juice, olive oil, honey, minced garlic, ground cumin, and black pepper until well combined.

2. Stir in the chopped cilantro.

3. Serve over your favorite salad or use as a marinade for poultry or fish. Store any leftovers in an airtight container in the refrigerator.

Nutritional Information (per serving):

- Calories: 70
- Protein: 0g
- Sodium: 1mg
- Potassium: 10mg
- Total Fat: 7g
- Saturated Fat: 1g
- Cholesterol: 0mg
- Carbohydrates: 2g
- Fiber: 0g

Marinated Cucumber Salad

Prep Time: 10 minutes + Marinating Time: 1 hour

Serving Size: 1/2 cup

Ingredients:

- 2 cups cucumber, thinly sliced
- 1/4 cup red onion, thinly sliced
- 1/4 cup vinegar, apple cider
- 1 tbsp olive oil
- 1 tsp sugar, or sugar substitute
- 1/4 tsp black pepper
- 1 tbsp dill, fresh, chopped

Instructions:

1. In a mixing bowl, combine cucumber and red onion.

2. In a small bowl, whisk together apple cider vinegar, olive oil, sugar, and black pepper to create the marinade.

3. Pour the marinade over the cucumber and onion. Toss to coat evenly.

4. Cover and refrigerate for at least 1 hour to allow flavors to meld. Sprinkle with fresh dill before serving.

Nutritional Information (per serving):

- Calories: 50
- Protein: 0.5g
- Sodium: 2mg
- Potassium: 115mg
- Total Fat: 3.5g
- Saturated Fat: 0.5g
- Cholesterol: 0mg
- Carbohydrates: 4g
- Fiber: 0.5g

Matilde's Tuna Salad

Prep Time: 15 minutes

Serving Size: 1/2 cup

Ingredients:

- 4 oz tuna, canned in water, drained
- 1/4 cup celery, finely chopped
- 1/4 cup apple, finely chopped
- 2 tbsp Greek yogurt, plain, non-fat
- 1 tbsp mayonnaise, low-fat
- 1 tsp lemon juice
- 1/4 tsp black pepper
- 1 tbsp parsley, fresh, chopped

Instructions:

1. In a bowl, mix the tuna, celery, and apple.

2. In a separate small bowl, combine Greek yogurt, mayonnaise, lemon juice, and black pepper to create a dressing.

3. Fold the dressing into the tuna mixture until well combined.

4. Chill in the refrigerator for at least 30 minutes before serving. Garnish with fresh parsley.

Nutritional Information (per serving):

- Calories: 100
- Protein: 14g
- Sodium: 180mg
- Potassium: 150mg
- Total Fat: 3g
- Saturated Fat: 0.5g
- Cholesterol: 30mg
- Carbohydrates: 4g
- Fiber: 1g

Mexican Coleslaw

Prep Time: 15 minutes Cooking Time: 0 minutes Serving Size: 1 cup

Ingredients:

- 4 cups shredded cabbage (mix of red and green for color and nutrients)
- 1 medium carrot, shredded
- 1/4 cup cilantro, chopped
- 1/4 cup green onions, thinly sliced
- 1 small jalapeño, seeded and finely chopped (optional)
- 2 tablespoons lime juice
- 1 tablespoon apple cider vinegar
- 1 tablespoon olive oil

- 1/4 teaspoon black pepper
- 1/2 teaspoon cumin (optional, for flavor)

Instructions:

1. In a large bowl, combine the shredded cabbage, carrot, cilantro, green onions, and jalapeño (if using).
2. In a small bowl, whisk together lime juice, apple cider vinegar, olive oil, black pepper, and cumin until well blended.
3. Pour the dressing over the cabbage mixture and toss to coat evenly.
4. Allow the coleslaw to sit for at least 10 minutes before serving, to let the flavors meld together.

Nutritional Information (per serving):

- Calories: 45
- Protein: 1g
- Sodium: 20mg
- Potassium: 120mg
- Total Fat: 2.5g
- Saturated Fat: 0.4g
- Cholesterol: 0mg
- Carbohydrates: 5g
- Fiber: 2g

Peach Basil Vinaigrette Dressing

Prep Time: 10 minutes Cooking Time: 0 minutes Serving Size: 2 tablespoons

Ingredients:

- 1 ripe peach, pitted and chopped
- 1/4 cup basil leaves, fresh
- 2 tablespoons white balsamic vinegar
- 1 tablespoon olive oil
- 1 teaspoon honey (optional, adjust based on dietary needs)
- 1/4 teaspoon black pepper
- 1/8 teaspoon salt (optional, can be omitted for lower sodium)

Instructions:

1. Combine the peach, basil, vinegar, olive oil, honey (if using), black pepper, and salt (if using) in a blender.
2. Blend until smooth. Taste and adjust seasoning as needed.
3. Store in an airtight container in the refrigerator for up to 5 days.

Nutritional Information (per serving):

- Calories: 35
- Protein: 0.2g
- Sodium: 15mg (without added salt)
- Potassium: 49mg
- Total Fat: 2.5g
- Saturated Fat: 0.4g
- Cholesterol: 0mg
- Carbohydrates: 3g
- Fiber: 0.5g

Pear and Cranberry Salad with Honey-Ginger Dressing

Prep Time: 20 minutes Cooking Time: 0 minutes Serving Size: 1 cup

Ingredients:

- 4 cups mixed greens (spinach, arugula, and lettuce)
- 1 ripe pear, cored and sliced
- 1/4 cup dried cranberries, low sugar or unsweetened
- 1/4 cup walnuts, chopped (optional, based on dietary phosphorus allowance)
- **Dressing:**
    - 2 tablespoons olive oil
    - 1 tablespoon lemon juice
    - 1 teaspoon honey
    - 1/2 teaspoon fresh ginger, grated
    - 1/8 teaspoon black pepper

Instructions:

1. In a large salad bowl, combine mixed greens, sliced pear, dried cranberries, and walnuts (if using).
2. In a small bowl, whisk together olive oil, lemon juice, honey, grated ginger, and black pepper for the dressing.
3. Drizzle the dressing over the salad and toss gently to combine.

Nutritional Information (per serving):

- Calories: 150
- Protein: 2g
- Sodium: 20mg
- Potassium: 200mg
- Total Fat: 8g
- Saturated Fat: 1g
- Cholesterol: 0mg
- Carbohydrates: 20g
- Fiber: 3g

Roasted Carrot and Cauliflower Salad

Prep Time: 15 minutes Cooking Time: 25 minutes Serving Size: 1 cup

Ingredients:

- 2 cups carrots, peeled and sliced
- 2 cups cauliflower florets
- 2 tablespoons olive oil
- 1/4 teaspoon black pepper
- 1/4 cup parsley, chopped
- **Dressing:**
    - 2 tablespoons lemon juice
    - 1 tablespoon olive oil
    - 1 teaspoon Dijon mustard
    - 1/4 teaspoon garlic powder

Instructions:

1. Preheat the oven to 425°F. Toss carrots and cauliflower with 2 tablespoons olive oil and black pepper. Spread on a baking sheet.
2. Roast for 25 minutes, stirring halfway through, until vegetables are tender and caramelized.
3. Prepare the dressing by whisking together lemon juice, 1 tablespoon olive oil, Dijon mustard, and garlic powder.

4. Toss the roasted vegetables with the dressing and parsley. Serve warm or at room temperature.

Nutritional Information (per serving):

- Calories: 120
- Protein: 2g
- Sodium: 45mg
- Potassium: 360mg
- Total Fat: 7g
- Saturated Fat: 1g
- Cholesterol: 0mg
- Carbohydrates: 13g
- Fiber: 4g

Roasted Vegetable Salad

Prep Time: 20 minutes Cooking Time: 30 minutes Serving Size: 1 cup

Ingredients:

- 1 red bell pepper, sliced
- 1 yellow bell pepper, sliced
- 1 zucchini, sliced
- 1 eggplant, cubed
- 2 tablespoons olive oil
- 1/4 teaspoon black pepper
- 2 cups mixed greens
- **Dressing:**
    - 2 tablespoons balsamic vinegar
    - 1 tablespoon olive oil
    - 1 teaspoon honey
    - 1/4 teaspoon dried oregano

Instructions:

1. Preheat the oven to 425°F. Toss the bell peppers, zucchini, and eggplant with olive oil and black pepper. Spread on a baking sheet.
2. Roast for 30 minutes, stirring occasionally, until vegetables are tender and have browned edges.
3. Whisk together balsamic vinegar, olive oil, honey, and oregano for the dressing.
4. Arrange mixed greens on a platter, top with roasted vegetables, and drizzle with dressing.

Nutritional Information (per serving):

- Calories: 130
- Protein: 2g
- Sodium: 30mg
- Potassium: 450mg
- Total Fat: 7g
- Saturated Fat: 1g
- Cholesterol: 0mg
- Carbohydrates: 16g
- Fiber: 5g

Tuna Pasta Salad

Prep Time: 20 minutes

Cooking Time: 10 minutes

Serving Size: 1 cup

Ingredients:

• 2 cups cooked whole wheat pasta (cooled)

• 1 can (4 ounces) no-salt-added tuna, drained and flaked

• 1/2 cup diced celery

• 1/4 cup chopped red bell pepper

• 1/4 cup shredded carrot

• 2 tablespoons chopped red onion

- 1/4 cup low-fat mayonnaise

- 1 tablespoon lemon juice

- 1 teaspoon dried dill

- 1/4 teaspoon black pepper

Instructions:

1. In a large bowl, combine the cooked pasta, tuna, celery, bell pepper, carrot, and red onion.

2. In a small bowl, whisk together the mayonnaise, lemon juice, dill, and black pepper.

3. Pour the dressing over the pasta mixture and toss to coat evenly.

4. Chill in the refrigerator for at least 1 hour before serving to allow flavors to meld.

Nutritional Information (per serving):

- Calories: 220

- Protein: 14g

- Sodium: 190mg

- Potassium: 300mg

- Total Fat: 4g

- Saturated Fat: 0.5g

- Cholesterol: 30mg

- Carbohydrates: 32g

- Fiber: 5g

Tuna Veggie Salad

Prep Time: 15 minutes

Serving Size: 1 cup

Ingredients:

- 1 can (4 ounces) no-salt-added tuna, drained and flaked

- 1 cup mixed greens

- 1/2 cup sliced cucumber

- 1/2 cup halved cherry tomatoes

- 1/4 cup diced avocado

- 1 tablespoon olive oil

- 2 teaspoons apple cider vinegar

- 1/4 teaspoon garlic powder

- 1/4 teaspoon black pepper

Instructions:

1. Arrange the mixed greens in a bowl. Top with tuna, cucumber, cherry tomatoes, and avocado.

2. In a small bowl, whisk together olive oil, apple cider vinegar, garlic powder, and black pepper.

3. Drizzle the dressing over the salad and gently toss to combine.

Nutritional Information (per serving):

- Calories: 200

- Protein: 14g

- Sodium: 180mg

- Potassium: 450mg

- Total Fat: 12g

- Saturated Fat: 2g

- Cholesterol: 30mg

- Carbohydrates: 8g

- Fiber: 4g

Watermelon and Cucumber Salad

Prep Time: 15 minutes

Serving Size: 1 cup

Ingredients:

• 2 cups diced watermelon

• 1 cup diced cucumber

• 1/4 cup thinly sliced red onion

• 2 tablespoons chopped fresh mint

• 1 tablespoon lime juice

• 1/8 teaspoon black pepper

Instructions:

1. In a large bowl, combine watermelon, cucumber, red onion, and fresh mint.

2. Drizzle with lime juice and sprinkle with black pepper.

3. Toss gently to combine and serve immediately.

Nutritional Information (per serving):

• Calories: 45

• Protein: 1g

• Sodium: 5mg

• Potassium: 170mg

• Total Fat: 0g

• Saturated Fat: 0g

• Cholesterol: 0mg

• Carbohydrates: 11g

• Fiber: 1g

White Egg Salad

Prep Time: 15 minutes

Cooking Time: 0 minutes (assuming pre-cooked egg whites)

Serving Size: 1/2 cup

Ingredients:

• 1 cup diced cooked egg whites

• 1/4 cup low-fat Greek yogurt

• 1 tablespoon chopped fresh dill

• 1/4 cup diced celery

• 1/4 teaspoon black pepper

• 1/4 teaspoon mustard powder

Instructions:

1. In a bowl, combine the cooked egg whites, Greek yogurt, dill, celery, black pepper, and mustard powder.

2. Mix until well combined and creamy.

3. Chill in the refrigerator before serving, or serve immediately on whole-grain toast or lettuce wraps.

Nutritional Information (per serving):

• Calories: 70

• Protein: 13g

• Sodium: 110mg

• Potassium: 180mg

• Total Fat: 1g

• Saturated Fat: 0g

• Cholesterol: 0mg

• Carbohydrates: 2g

• Fiber: 0g

SEAFOOD

Baked Trout with Lemon and Dill

Prep Time: 10 minutes Cooking Time: 15 minutes Serving Size: 1 filet

Ingredients:

- 4 trout filets (about 6 ounces each)
- 2 tablespoons olive oil
- 1 lemon, thinly sliced
- 2 tablespoons fresh dill, chopped
- 1/4 teaspoon black pepper

Instructions:

1. Preheat the oven to 375°F. Line a baking sheet with parchment paper.
2. Place trout filets on the prepared baking sheet. Drizzle each filet with olive oil.
3. Top each filet with lemon slices and sprinkle with dill and black pepper.
4. Bake in the preheated oven for about 15 minutes or until the trout is opaque and flakes easily with a fork.

Nutritional Information (per serving):

- Calories: 280
- Protein: 35g
- Sodium: 70mg
- Potassium: 560mg
- Total Fat: 15g
- Saturated Fat: 3g
- Cholesterol: 88mg
- Carbohydrates: 1g
- Fiber: 0.2g

Broiled Cod with Cucumber Sauce

Prep Time: 15 minutes Cooking Time: 10 minutes Serving Size: 1 filet

Ingredients:

- 4 cod filets (about 6 ounces each)
- 1 tablespoon olive oil
- 1/4 teaspoon black pepper
- 1 cup Greek yogurt, low-fat
- 1 cucumber, seeded and finely diced
- 1 tablespoon fresh dill, chopped
- 1 tablespoon lemon juice
- 1/4 teaspoon garlic powder

Instructions:

1. Preheat the broiler. Line a baking sheet with aluminum foil and lightly grease with olive oil.
2. Place cod filets on the prepared baking sheet. Brush each filet with olive oil and sprinkle with black pepper.
3. Broil for about 10 minutes or until the cod is opaque and flakes easily with a fork.
4. While the cod is broiling, mix Greek yogurt, cucumber, dill, lemon juice, and garlic powder in a bowl to create the sauce.
5. Serve each cod filet with a generous dollop of cucumber sauce on top.

Nutritional Information (per serving):

- Calories: 220
- Protein: 32g
- Sodium: 95mg
- Potassium: 780mg
- Total Fat: 5g
- Saturated Fat: 1g
- Cholesterol: 60mg
- Carbohydrates: 5g
- Fiber: 0.5g

Broiled Haddock with Cucumber Salsa

Prep Time: 20 minutes Cooking Time: 12 minutes Serving Size: 1 filet

Ingredients:

- 4 haddock filets (about 6 ounces each)
- 2 teaspoons olive oil
- 1/4 teaspoon black pepper
- 1 cucumber, seeded and diced
- 1/2 red bell pepper, diced
- 1/4 cup red onion, finely chopped
- 2 tablespoons fresh cilantro, chopped
- 1 tablespoon lime juice
- 1/4 teaspoon garlic powder

Instructions:

1. Preheat the broiler. Line a broiling pan with foil and lightly brush with olive oil.
2. Season haddock filets with black pepper and brush with olive oil. Place on the prepared pan.
3. Broil for 10-12 minutes, or until the fish is opaque and flakes easily with a fork.
4. While the fish is broiling, combine cucumber, red bell pepper, red onion, cilantro, lime juice, and garlic powder in a bowl to make the salsa.
5. Serve the broiled haddock topped with the fresh cucumber salsa.

Nutritional Information (per serving):

- Calories: 200
- Protein: 34g
- Sodium: 85mg
- Potassium: 650mg
- Total Fat: 4g
- Saturated Fat: 1g
- Cholesterol: 95mg
- Carbohydrates: 6g
- Fiber: 1g

Cilantro-Lime Cod

Prep Time: 15 minutes Cooking Time: 12 minutes Serving Size: 1 filet

Ingredients:

- 4 cod filets (about 6 ounces each)
- 2 tablespoons olive oil
- 1/4 cup fresh cilantro, finely chopped
- 2 tablespoons lime juice
- 1/4 teaspoon black pepper
- Lime slices for garnish

Instructions:

1. Preheat the oven to 400°F. Line a baking dish with parchment paper.
2. In a small bowl, mix together olive oil, cilantro, lime juice, and black pepper.

3. Place cod filets in the baking dish and brush each filet with the cilantro-lime mixture.

4. Bake in the preheated oven for 12 minutes, or until the fish flakes easily with a fork.

5. Garnish with lime slices before serving.

Nutritional Information (per serving):

- Calories: 220
- Protein: 33g
- Sodium: 90mg
- Potassium: 740mg
- Total Fat: 10g
- Saturated Fat: 1.5g
- Cholesterol: 65mg
- Carbohydrates: 1g
- Fiber: 0g

Citrus Salmon

Prep Time: 15 minutes Cooking Time: 15 minutes Serving Size: 1 filet

Ingredients:

- 4 salmon filets (about 6 ounces each)
- 2 tablespoons olive oil
- 1 orange, sliced
- 1 lemon, sliced
- 1 lime, sliced
- 1/4 teaspoon black pepper
- Fresh dill for garnish

Instructions:

1. Preheat the oven to 375°F. Line a baking sheet with parchment paper.

2. Arrange the salmon filets on the baking sheet and drizzle with olive oil. Season with black pepper.

3. Top each filet with orange, lemon, and lime slices.

4. Bake for 15 minutes, or until the salmon is opaque and flakes easily with a fork.

5. Garnish with fresh dill before serving.

Nutritional Information (per serving):

- Calories: 300
- Protein: 34g
- Sodium: 75mg
- Potassium: 830mg
- Total Fat: 17g
- Saturated Fat: 2.5g
- Cholesterol: 88mg
- Carbohydrates: 5g
- Fiber: 1g

Crab Cakes

Prep Time: 25 minutes

Cooking Time: 10 minutes

Serving Size: 2 cakes

Ingredients:

- 8 oz crabmeat, fresh or canned, drained and shell pieces removed
- 1/4 cup red bell pepper, finely chopped
- 2 tablespoons scallions, thinly sliced
- 1/4 cup whole wheat breadcrumbs
- 1 egg, beaten
- 2 tablespoons Greek yogurt, plain
- 1 teaspoon Dijon mustard
- 1/4 teaspoon ground black pepper

- 1 tablespoon olive oil for cooking

Instructions:

1. In a large bowl, combine crabmeat, red bell pepper, scallions, and breadcrumbs.
2. In a separate small bowl, whisk together the egg, Greek yogurt, Dijon mustard, and black pepper until smooth.
3. Fold the wet ingredients into the crab mixture until well combined.
4. Form the mixture into 4 cakes and set aside on a plate.
5. Heat olive oil in a non-stick skillet over medium heat. Cook the crab cakes for about 5 minutes on each side, until golden brown and heated through.

Nutritional Information (per serving):

- Calories: 190
- Protein: 23g
- Sodium: 380mg
- Potassium: 340mg
- Total Fat: 7g
- Saturated Fat: 1g
- Cholesterol: 95mg
- Carbohydrates: 9g
- Fiber: 1g

Creamy Baked Fish

Prep Time: 15 minutes

Cooking Time: 20 minutes

Serving Size: 1 fillet

Ingredients:

- 4 white fish fillets (such as cod or tilapia), about 6 ounces each
- 1/2 cup Greek yogurt, plain
- 2 tablespoons lemon juice
- 1 tablespoon fresh dill, chopped
- 1/4 teaspoon garlic powder
- 1/4 teaspoon ground black pepper
- Lemon slices and fresh dill for garnish

Instructions:

1. Preheat the oven to 375°F. Arrange fish fillets in a single layer in a greased baking dish.
2. In a small bowl, mix together Greek yogurt, lemon juice, chopped dill, garlic powder, and black pepper.
3. Spread the yogurt mixture evenly over the fish fillets.
4. Bake in the preheated oven for 20 minutes, or until the fish flakes easily with a fork.
5. Garnish with lemon slices and additional fresh dill before serving.

Nutritional Information (per serving):

- Calories: 140
- Protein: 26g
- Sodium: 125mg
- Potassium: 520mg
- Total Fat: 2g

- Saturated Fat: 0.5g

- Cholesterol: 60mg

- Carbohydrates: 3g

- Fiber: 0g

Easy Shrimp in Garlic Sauce

Prep Time: 10 minutes

Cooking Time: 10 minutes

Serving Size: 1 cup

Ingredients:

- 1 lb shrimp, peeled and deveined

- 2 tablespoons olive oil

- 3 cloves garlic, minced

- 1/4 cup low-sodium chicken broth

- 1 tablespoon lemon juice

- 1/4 teaspoon red pepper flakes

- 2 tablespoons fresh parsley, chopped

- 1/4 teaspoon ground black pepper

Instructions:

1. Heat olive oil in a large skillet over medium heat. Add garlic and sauté until fragrant, about 1 minute.

2. Add shrimp and cook until pink and opaque, about 2-3 minutes per side.

3. Pour in chicken broth and lemon juice, sprinkle with red pepper flakes and black pepper. Bring to a simmer.

4. Cook for an additional 2 minutes, or until the sauce has slightly thickened.

5. Remove from heat, stir in chopped parsley, and serve.

Nutritional Information (per serving):

- Calories: 160

- Protein: 24g

- Sodium: 210mg

- Potassium: 200mg

- Total Fat: 6g

- Saturated Fat: 1g

- Cholesterol: 180mg

- Carbohydrates: 3g

- Fiber: 0g

Fish Fry with Seasoned Rice

Prep Time: 15 minutes

Cooking Time: 30 minutes

Serving Size: 1 fillet and 1/2 cup rice

Ingredients for Fish:

- 4 white fish fillets (such as haddock), about 6 ounces each

- 1/4 cup almond flour

- 1/4 teaspoon garlic powder

- 1/4 teaspoon ground black pepper

- 2 tablespoons olive oil

Ingredients for Seasoned Rice:

- 1 cup brown rice, uncooked

- 2 cups water

- 1 bay leaf

- 1/4 teaspoon turmeric

- 1/4 teaspoon garlic powder

- 1/4 teaspoon onion powder

Instructions:

1. Combine almond flour, garlic powder, and black pepper in a shallow dish. Dredge fish fillets in the mixture.

2. Heat olive oil in a large skillet over medium heat. Add fish fillets and cook

for 4-5 minutes on each side, until golden brown and fish flakes easily with a fork.

3. For the rice, combine rice, water, bay leaf, turmeric, garlic powder, and onion powder in a medium saucepan. Bring to a boil, then reduce heat to low, cover, and simmer for 25 minutes, or until water is absorbed.

4. Remove bay leaf before serving. Serve fish fillets with a side of seasoned rice.

Nutritional Information (per serving for fish and rice):

- Calories: 320
- Protein: 28g
- Sodium: 75mg
- Potassium: 450mg
- Total Fat: 10g
- Saturated Fat: 1.5g
- Cholesterol: 55mg
- Carbohydrates: 28g
- Fiber: 3g

Fish Tacos

Prep Time: 20 minutes
Cooking Time: 10 minutes
Serving Size: 2 tacos
Ingredients:

- 4 white fish fillets (such as tilapia), about 3 ounces each
- 1 tablespoon olive oil
- 1 teaspoon chili powder
- 1/2 teaspoon ground cumin
- 1/4 teaspoon garlic powder
- 8 small corn tortillas
- 1 cup cabbage, shredded
- 1/2 cup Greek yogurt, plain
- 1 lime, cut into wedges
- Fresh cilantro for garnish

Instructions:

1. Preheat the grill or grill pan over medium heat. Brush fish fillets with olive oil and season with chili powder, cumin, and garlic powder.

2. Grill fish for about 4-5 minutes on each side, until cooked through and easily flaked with a fork.

3. Warm tortillas on the grill for about 30 seconds on each side.

4. Divide fish among tortillas and top with shredded cabbage.

5. Serve with a dollop of Greek yogurt, a squeeze of lime, and garnished with fresh cilantro.

Nutritional Information (per serving):

- Calories: 220
- Protein: 23g
- Sodium: 85mg
- Potassium: 360mg
- Total Fat: 6g
- Saturated Fat: 1g
- Cholesterol: 45mg
- Carbohydrates: 22g
- Fiber: 3g

Grilled Mexican Swordfish Fillets

Prep Time: 25 minutes

Cooking Time: 10 minutes

Serving Size: 4 ounces (about 114 grams) per fillet

Ingredients:

- 4 swordfish fillets (6 ounces each)
- 2 tablespoons olive oil
- 1 tablespoon lime juice
- 1 teaspoon garlic, minced
- 1 teaspoon chili powder (low sodium)
- 1/4 teaspoon ground cumin
- Fresh cilantro, chopped (for garnish)
- Lime wedges (for serving)

Instructions:

1. In a small bowl, whisk together olive oil, lime juice, minced garlic, chili powder, and ground cumin to create a marinade.
2. Place swordfish fillets in a shallow dish and pour the marinade over them, ensuring each fillet is well-coated. Marinate in the refrigerator for 15 to 20 minutes.
3. Preheat the grill to medium-high heat. Remove the fillets from the marinade, discarding any excess marinade.
4. Grill the fillets for about 5 minutes on each side or until the fish flakes easily with a fork.
5. Garnish with chopped cilantro and serve with lime wedges on the side.

Nutritional Information (per serving):

- Calories: 280
- Protein: 34g
- Sodium: 95mg
- Potassium: 450mg
- Total Fat: 15g
- Saturated Fat: 3g
- Cholesterol: 90mg
- Carbohydrates: 1g
- Fiber: 0g

Grilled Salmon

Prep Time: 20 minutes

Cooking Time: 15 minutes

Serving Size: 4 ounces (about 114 grams) per piece

Ingredients:

- 4 salmon fillets (6 ounces each)
- 2 tablespoons lemon juice
- 2 teaspoons olive oil
- 1 teaspoon dried dill weed
- 1/4 teaspoon black pepper
- Lemon slices (for garnish)

Instructions:

1. Preheat the grill to medium heat.
2. In a small bowl, mix together lemon juice, olive oil, dill weed, and black pepper.
3. Brush the mixture over both sides of the salmon fillets.
4. Place the salmon on the grill, skin side down, and cook for 6-8 minutes. Flip carefully and grill for another 6-7

minutes or until the salmon is opaque throughout.

5. Garnish with lemon slices before serving.

Nutritional Information (per serving):

- Calories: 280
- Protein: 34g
- Sodium: 75mg
- Potassium: 830mg
- Total Fat: 14g
- Saturated Fat: 2g
- Cholesterol: 85mg
- Carbohydrates: 1g
- Fiber: 0g

Salmon Steaks with Herb Dressing

Prep Time: 15 minutes

Cooking Time: 10 minutes

Serving Size: 4 ounces of salmon per person

Ingredients:

- 4 salmon steaks (about 6 ounces each)
- 2 tablespoons olive oil
- 1 teaspoon garlic, minced
- Juice of 1 lemon
- 2 tablespoons fresh dill, chopped
- 2 tablespoons fresh parsley, chopped
- Black pepper to taste

Instructions:

1. Preheat the grill or oven broiler to medium-high heat. Lightly oil the grill grate or a baking sheet.

2. Mix olive oil, garlic, lemon juice, dill, parsley, and black pepper in a small bowl. Set aside half of the mixture for serving.

3. Brush both sides of the salmon steaks with the remaining herb mixture.

4. Grill or broil the salmon for about 5 minutes per side, or until the fish flakes easily with a fork.

5. Serve the salmon steaks with the reserved herb dressing drizzled on top.

Nutritional Information (per serving):

- Calories: 280
- Protein: 34g
- Sodium: 75mg
- Potassium: 830mg
- Total Fat: 15g
- Saturated Fat: 2.5g
- Cholesterol: 90mg
- Carbohydrates: 1g
- Fiber: 0g

Sheet Pan Salmon and Green Beans

Prep Time: 10 minutes

Cooking Time: 20 minutes

Serving Size: 4 ounces of salmon and ½ cup green beans per person

Ingredients:

- 4 salmon fillets (about 6 ounces each)
- 2 cups green beans, trimmed
- 2 tablespoons olive oil
- 1 teaspoon garlic, minced

- Lemon slices
- Black pepper to taste

Instructions:

1. Preheat the oven to 400°F. Line a sheet pan with parchment paper.
2. Toss green beans with half the olive oil and garlic. Spread them around the edges of the sheet pan.
3. Place salmon fillets in the center of the pan. Drizzle with remaining olive oil and season with black pepper. Top with lemon slices.
4. Roast for 18-20 minutes, or until the salmon is cooked through and green beans are tender.
5. Serve immediately.

Nutritional Information (per serving):

- Calories: 295
- Protein: 35g
- Sodium: 60mg
- Potassium: 900mg
- Total Fat: 16g
- Saturated Fat: 2.5g
- Cholesterol: 85mg
- Carbohydrates: 5g
- Fiber: 2g

Shrimp and Asparagus Linguini

Prep Time: 20 minutes

Cooking Time: 15 minutes

Serving Size: 1 cup cooked pasta with shrimp and asparagus

Ingredients:

- 8 ounces whole wheat linguini
- 1 pound shrimp, peeled and deveined
- 2 cups asparagus, cut into 1-inch pieces
- 2 tablespoons olive oil
- 1 teaspoon garlic, minced
- 1 lemon, juice and zest
- Black pepper to taste

Instructions:

1. Cook linguini according to package instructions. Drain and set aside.
2. In a large skillet, heat olive oil over medium heat. Add garlic and sauté for 1 minute.
3. Add shrimp and asparagus to the skillet. Cook until shrimp are pink and asparagus is tender, about 5-7 minutes.
4. Toss the cooked linguini with the shrimp and asparagus mixture. Add lemon juice, zest, and black pepper. Combine well.
5. Serve warm.

Nutritional Information (per serving):

- Calories: 320
- Protein: 28g
- Sodium: 190mg
- Potassium: 300mg
- Total Fat: 8g
- Saturated Fat: 1g

- Cholesterol: 182mg
- Carbohydrates: 35g
- Fiber: 6g

Sole with Tarragon Cream Sauce

Prep Time: 10 minutes

Cooking Time: 20 minutes

Serving Size: 1 fillet with sauce

Ingredients:

- 4 sole fillets (about 6 ounces each)
- 1 tablespoon olive oil
- 1 cup low-sodium vegetable broth
- 1 teaspoon fresh tarragon, chopped
- 1/2 cup heavy cream
- 1 teaspoon Dijon mustard
- Black pepper to taste

Instructions:

1. Heat olive oil in a large skillet over medium heat. Add sole fillets and cook for about 2-3 minutes on each side, or until cooked through. Remove from skillet and keep warm.
2. In the same skillet, add vegetable broth and tarragon. Bring to a simmer and reduce by half.
3. Stir in heavy cream and Dijon mustard. Simmer until the sauce thickens slightly.
4. Season with black pepper. Serve the sauce over the sole fillets.

Nutritional Information (per serving):

- Calories: 225
- Protein: 23g
- Sodium: 125mg
- Potassium: 350mg
- Total Fat: 13g
- Saturated Fat: 5g
- Cholesterol: 85mg
- Carbohydrates: 3g
- Fiber: 0g

South of the Border Shrimp Cocktail

Prep Time: 20 minutes

Cooking Time: 5 minutes

Serving Size: 1 cup

Ingredients:

- 1 pound cooked shrimp, peeled and deveined
- 1 cup cucumber, diced
- 1/2 cup celery, diced
- 1/4 cup red onion, finely chopped
- 1/2 cup tomato, diced
- 1/4 cup fresh cilantro, chopped
- Juice of 2 limes
- 1 tablespoon olive oil
- 1/2 teaspoon chili powder (adjust to taste)
- Black pepper to taste

Instructions:

1. In a large bowl, combine the cooked shrimp, cucumber, celery, red onion, tomato, and cilantro.
2. In a small bowl, whisk together lime juice, olive oil, chili powder, and black pepper.

3. Pour the dressing over the shrimp mixture and stir gently to combine.

4. Chill in the refrigerator for at least 1 hour before serving to allow flavors to meld.

Nutritional Information (per serving):

- Calories: 180
- Protein: 24g
- Sodium: 200mg
- Potassium: 350mg
- Total Fat: 5g
- Saturated Fat: 0.7g
- Cholesterol: 182mg
- Carbohydrates: 8g
- Fiber: 2g

Spicy Seafood Étouffée

Prep Time: 15 minutes

Cooking Time: 30 minutes

Serving Size: 1 cup

Ingredients:

- 1 tablespoon olive oil
- 1/2 cup onion, diced
- 1/2 cup bell pepper, diced
- 1/2 cup celery, diced
- 2 cloves garlic, minced
- 1 tablespoon no-salt-added tomato paste
- 1 cup low-sodium vegetable broth
- 1 teaspoon paprika
- 1/2 teaspoon cayenne pepper (adjust to taste)
- 1 pound mixed seafood (shrimp, scallops, crab meat)
- 1 tablespoon fresh parsley, chopped
- Black pepper to taste

Instructions:

1. Heat olive oil in a large skillet over medium heat. Add onion, bell pepper, celery, and garlic. Cook until vegetables are soft, about 5 minutes.

2. Stir in tomato paste, vegetable broth, paprika, and cayenne pepper. Bring to a simmer.

3. Add the seafood to the skillet. Cover and simmer until seafood is cooked through, about 10-15 minutes.

4. Garnish with parsley and season with black pepper to taste.

5. Serve hot.

Nutritional Information (per serving):

- Calories: 200
- Protein: 25g
- Sodium: 250mg
- Potassium: 450mg
- Total Fat: 6g
- Saturated Fat: 1g
- Cholesterol: 150mg
- Carbohydrates: 10g
- Fiber: 2g

Thai Pineapple Shrimp and Jasmine Rice

Prep Time: 15 minutes

Cooking Time: 20 minutes

Serving Size: 1 cup cooked rice with shrimp mixture

Ingredients:

- 1 cup jasmine rice
- 1 tablespoon olive oil
- 1 pound shrimp, peeled and deveined
- 1 cup pineapple, diced
- 1/2 cup red bell pepper, diced
- 1/4 cup low-sodium soy sauce
- 1 tablespoon ginger, minced
- 1 clove garlic, minced
- Juice of 1 lime
- 1 tablespoon fresh basil, chopped

Instructions:

1. Cook jasmine rice according to package instructions and set aside.
2. Heat olive oil in a large skillet over medium-high heat. Add shrimp and cook until pink, about 3 minutes per side. Remove shrimp from skillet.
3. In the same skillet, add pineapple and red bell pepper. Cook until just tender, about 5 minutes.
4. Return shrimp to skillet. Add soy sauce, ginger, garlic, and lime juice. Cook for an additional 2 minutes.
5. Stir in fresh basil just before serving.
6. Serve the shrimp and pineapple mixture over jasmine rice.

Nutritional Information (per serving):

- Calories: 320
- Protein: 25g
- Sodium: 600mg
- Potassium: 300mg
- Total Fat: 5g
- Saturated Fat: 0.8g
- Cholesterol: 172mg
- Carbohydrates: 45g
- Fiber: 2g

Tuna Ceviche

Prep Time: 20 minutes (plus chilling time)

Cooking Time: 0 minutes

Serving Size: 1/2 cup

Ingredients:

- 1 pound fresh tuna, diced
- Juice of 3 limes
- 1/4 cup red onion, finely chopped
- 1/4 cup cucumber, diced
- 1/4 cup tomato, diced
- 1 tablespoon cilantro, chopped
- 1 avocado, diced
- Black pepper to taste

Instructions:

1. In a glass bowl, combine the diced tuna and lime juice. Ensure the tuna is completely covered by the juice. Chill in the refrigerator for at least 2 hours.
2. Drain the lime juice from the tuna. Add red onion, cucumber, tomato, cilantro,

and avocado to the bowl with the tuna. Gently mix.

3. Season with black pepper to taste.

4. Serve chilled.

Nutritional Information (per serving):

- Calories: 220
- Protein: 27g
- Sodium: 45mg
- Potassium: 500mg
- Total Fat: 9g
- Saturated Fat: 1.5g
- Cholesterol: 45mg
- Carbohydrates: 9g
- Fiber: 3g

Tuna Noodle Casserole for Two

Prep Time: 10 minutes

Cooking Time: 20 minutes

Serving Size: 1/2 of the casserole

Ingredients:

- 4 ounces whole wheat noodles
- 1 can (6 ounces) no-salt-added tuna, drained
- 1 cup mushrooms, sliced
- 1/2 cup peas, frozen
- 1/2 cup low-sodium vegetable broth
- 1/2 cup Greek yogurt, plain
- 1 teaspoon Dijon mustard
- Black pepper to taste
- 1 tablespoon whole wheat breadcrumbs

Instructions:

1. Preheat oven to 375°F. Cook noodles according to package instructions, drain and set aside.

2. In a mixing bowl, combine tuna, mushrooms, peas, vegetable broth, Greek yogurt, Dijon mustard, and black pepper.

3. Gently fold in cooked noodles until well combined.

4. Transfer the mixture to a baking dish. Sprinkle breadcrumbs on top.

5. Bake for 20 minutes or until the top is golden and crispy.

6. Serve warm.

Nutritional Information (per serving):

- Calories: 350
- Protein: 28g
- Sodium: 200mg
- Potassium: 450mg
- Total Fat: 6g
- Saturated Fat: 1g
- Cholesterol: 30mg
- Carbohydrates: 45g
- Fiber: 6g

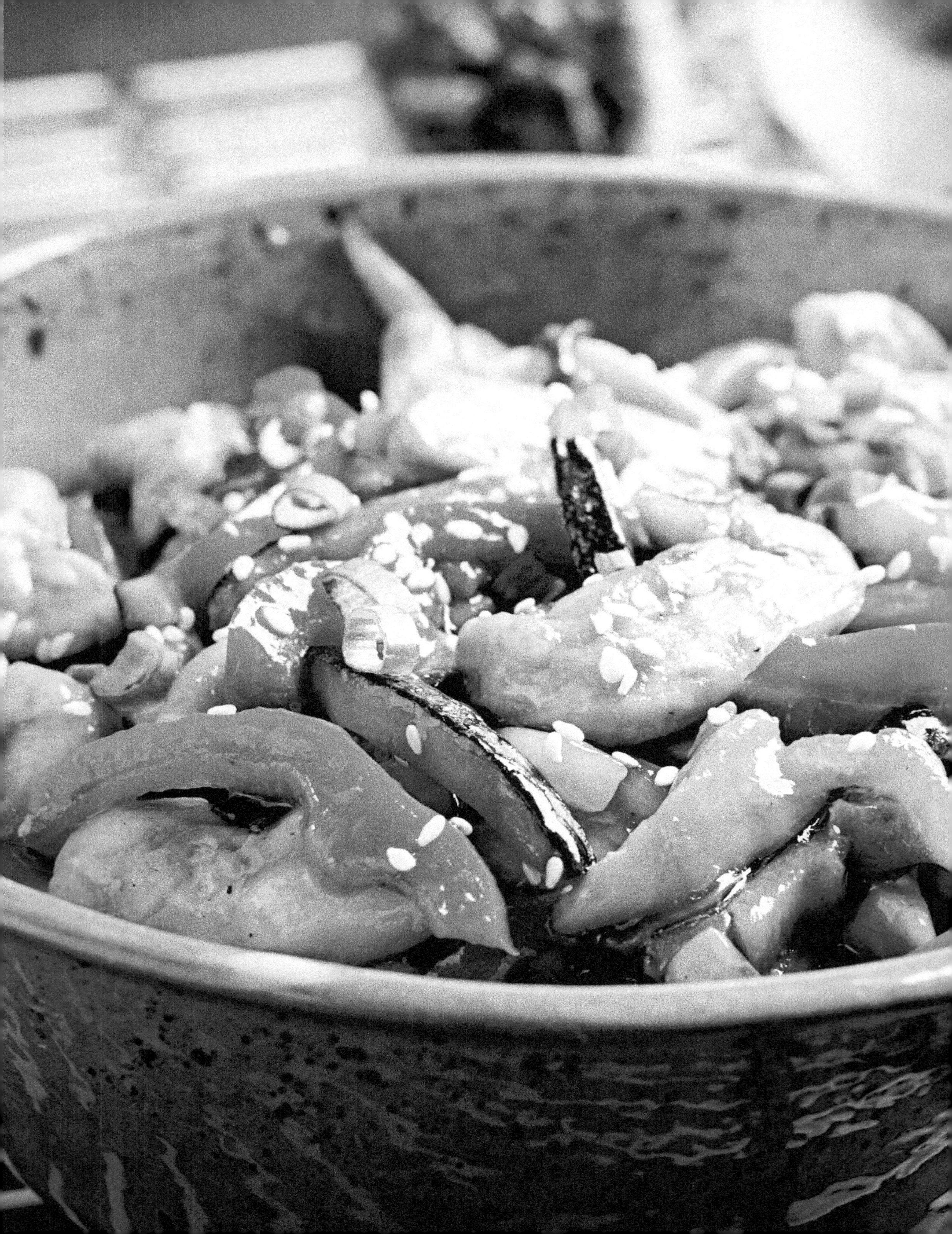

CHICKEN AND TURKEY

Asian-Style Turkey Bowls

Prep Time: 20 minutes

Cooking Time: 20 minutes

Serving Size: 1 bowl

Ingredients:

- 1 pound ground turkey, lean
- 2 tablespoons olive oil
- 1 cup brown rice, cooked
- 1 cup carrots, shredded
- 1 cup zucchini, shredded
- 1/2 cup low-sodium soy sauce
- 1 tablespoon ginger, minced
- 2 cloves garlic, minced
- 1 teaspoon honey
- 2 green onions, sliced for garnish

Instructions:

1. Cook the brown rice according to package instructions and set aside.
2. Heat olive oil in a large skillet over medium heat. Add the ground turkey and cook until browned, breaking it into small pieces as it cooks.
3. Add the shredded carrots and zucchini to the skillet. Cook for an additional 5 minutes, or until vegetables are tender.
4. In a small bowl, whisk together low-sodium soy sauce, ginger, garlic, and honey. Pour this mixture over the turkey and vegetables in the skillet. Stir to combine and cook for another 5 minutes to allow the flavors to meld.
5. Serve the turkey and vegetable mixture over the cooked brown rice. Garnish with sliced green onions.

Nutritional Information (per serving):

- Calories: 350
- Protein: 25g
- Sodium: 300mg
- Potassium: 650mg
- Total Fat: 12g
- Saturated Fat: 2g
- Cholesterol: 55mg
- Carbohydrates: 35g
- Fiber: 4g

Cabbage Rolls Made with Turkey

Prep Time: 30 minutes

Cooking Time: 1 hour

Serving Size: 2 rolls

Ingredients:

- 8 large cabbage leaves
- 1 pound ground turkey, lean
- 1 cup cooked quinoa
- 1/4 cup onion, minced
- 1 clove garlic, minced
- 1 teaspoon olive oil
- 1 cup low-sodium tomato sauce
- 1 teaspoon dried oregano
- 1 teaspoon dried basil

- Black pepper to taste

Instructions:

1. Preheat oven to 350°F.
2. Blanch cabbage leaves in boiling water for 2 minutes or until pliable. Drain and set aside.
3. In a bowl, combine ground turkey, cooked quinoa, onion, garlic, oregano, basil, and black pepper.
4. Place a portion of the turkey mixture into the center of each cabbage leaf. Fold in the sides and roll up tightly.
5. Place the rolls seam-side down in a baking dish. Drizzle with olive oil and pour tomato sauce over the rolls.
6. Cover and bake for about 1 hour or until the meat is cooked through.
7. Serve hot.

Nutritional Information (per serving):

- Calories: 240
- Protein: 28g
- Sodium: 200mg
- Potassium: 500mg
- Total Fat: 8g
- Saturated Fat: 1.5g
- Cholesterol: 65mg
- Carbohydrates: 18g
- Fiber: 4g

Caribbean Curry Turkey

Prep Time: 15 minutes

Cooking Time: 30 minutes

Serving Size: 1 cup

Ingredients:

- 1 pound turkey breast, cut into cubes
- 1 tablespoon olive oil
- 1 onion, diced
- 1 bell pepper, diced
- 2 cloves garlic, minced
- 1 tablespoon curry powder (adjust to taste)
- 1 cup low-sodium chicken broth
- 1 teaspoon thyme
- 1 teaspoon paprika
- Black pepper to taste

Instructions:

1. Heat olive oil in a large skillet over medium heat. Add onion, bell pepper, and garlic. Cook until softened, about 5 minutes.
2. Add the turkey cubes to the skillet. Cook until browned on all sides.
3. Sprinkle curry powder, thyme, paprika, and black pepper over the turkey and vegetables. Stir to coat evenly.
4. Pour in the chicken broth. Bring to a simmer, then reduce heat, cover, and let cook for 20 minutes, or until the turkey is cooked through and tender.
5. Serve hot, ideally with a side of cooked cauliflower rice.

- Calories: 220
- Protein: 27g
- Sodium: 200mg
- Potassium: 450mg
- Total Fat: 7g
- Saturated Fat: 1g
- Cholesterol: 55mg
- Carbohydrates: 9g
- Fiber: 2g

Chicken and Apple Curry

Prep Time: 15 minutes

Cooking Time: 25 minutes

Serving Size: 1 cup

Ingredients:

- 1 pound chicken breast, cubed
- 1 tablespoon olive oil
- 1 onion, diced
- 2 apples, peeled and diced
- 2 teaspoons curry powder (adjust to taste)
- 1 cup low-sodium chicken broth
- 1/2 cup Greek yogurt, plain
- Black pepper to taste

Instructions:

1. Heat olive oil in a large skillet over medium heat. Add the chicken cubes and cook until browned. Remove chicken and set aside.
2. In the same skillet, add the onion and apples. Cook until the onion is translucent and apples are slightly soft.
3. Return the chicken to the skillet. Add curry powder and stir to coat the chicken and apples evenly.
4. Pour in the chicken broth and bring to a simmer. Cook for 15 minutes, or until the chicken is cooked through.
5. Remove from heat and stir in Greek yogurt. Season with black pepper to taste.
6. Serve hot, accompanied by cooked brown rice or quinoa.

Nutritional Information (per serving):

- Calories: 260
- Protein: 28g
- Sodium: 200mg
- Potassium: 600mg
- Total Fat: 8g
- Saturated Fat: 1.5g
- Cholesterol: 70mg
- Carbohydrates: 18g
- Fiber: 3g

Chicken and Rice Casserole

Prep Time: 10 minutes

Cooking Time: 45 minutes

Serving Size: 1/2 of the casserole

Ingredients:

- 2 chicken breasts, diced
- 1 cup brown rice, uncooked
- 2 cups low-sodium chicken broth
- 1 cup mushrooms, sliced
- 1/2 cup peas
- 1/2 cup carrots, diced

- 1 teaspoon olive oil
- 1 teaspoon garlic powder
- 1 teaspoon onion powder
- Black pepper to taste

Instructions:

1. Preheat oven to 375°F.
2. In a large bowl, combine all ingredients and mix well.
3. Transfer the mixture to a baking dish. Cover with aluminum foil.
4. Bake for 45 minutes, or until the rice is cooked and the chicken is tender.
5. Remove foil and bake for an additional 5 minutes to slightly crisp the top.
6. Serve hot.

Nutritional Information (per serving):

- Calories: 320
- Protein: 30g
- Sodium: 200mg
- Potassium: 600mg
- Total Fat: 6g
- Saturated Fat: 1g
- Cholesterol: 75mg
- Carbohydrates: 35g
- Fiber: 4g

Chicken in Rosemary-Garlic Sauce

Prep Time: 15 minutes

Cooking Time: 25 minutes

Serving Size: 1 breast

Ingredients:

- 4 chicken breasts, boneless and skinless
- 2 tablespoons olive oil
- 4 cloves garlic, minced
- 1 tablespoon fresh rosemary, chopped
- 1 cup low-sodium chicken broth
- Black pepper to taste

Instructions:

1. Heat olive oil in a large skillet over medium heat. Add garlic and rosemary, sautéing until fragrant, about 1 minute.
2. Add chicken breasts to the skillet, cooking until golden on both sides, approximately 3-4 minutes per side.
3. Pour low-sodium chicken broth over the chicken, covering the skillet with a lid. Let simmer for 15-20 minutes, or until the chicken is cooked through.
4. Serve the chicken topped with the rosemary-garlic sauce from the skillet.

Nutritional Information (per serving):

- Calories: 220
- Protein: 26g
- Sodium: 150mg
- Potassium: 370mg
- Total Fat: 10g
- Saturated Fat: 1.5g
- Cholesterol: 75mg
- Carbohydrates: 2g
- Fiber: 0.5g

Chicken in Wine Sauce

Prep Time: 20 minutes

Cooking Time: 30 minutes

Serving Size: 1 breast

Ingredients:

- 4 chicken breasts, boneless and skinless
- 1 tablespoon olive oil
- 1/2 cup dry white wine (or low-sodium chicken broth for a non-alcoholic version)
- 1 cup mushrooms, sliced
- 1 onion, chopped
- 2 cloves garlic, minced
- 1 teaspoon thyme
- Black pepper to taste

Instructions:

1. In a large skillet, heat olive oil over medium-high heat. Add chicken breasts, cooking until each side is golden brown, about 3 minutes per side. Remove chicken and set aside.
2. In the same skillet, add mushrooms, onion, and garlic. Sauté until softened, about 5 minutes.
3. Return chicken to the skillet. Add white wine (or chicken broth), thyme, and black pepper. Cover and simmer for 20 minutes, or until the chicken is cooked through.
4. Serve the chicken with the mushroom and wine sauce spooned over the top.

Nutritional Information (per serving):

- Calories: 230
- Protein: 27g
- Sodium: 60mg
- Potassium: 400mg
- Total Fat: 7g
- Saturated Fat: 1g
- Cholesterol: 75mg
- Carbohydrates: 5g
- Fiber: 1g

Chicken with Apples, Carrots, and Grains

Prep Time: 20 minutes

Cooking Time: 30 minutes

Serving Size: 1 portion

Ingredients:

- 4 chicken breasts, boneless and skinless
- 2 tablespoons olive oil
- 2 apples, cored and sliced
- 2 carrots, sliced
- 1 cup mixed grains (quinoa and wild rice), cooked
- 1 teaspoon cinnamon
- 1 cup low-sodium vegetable broth
- Black pepper to taste

Instructions:

1. Preheat oven to 375°F.
2. In a large skillet, heat 1 tablespoon olive oil over medium heat. Add chicken breasts, cooking until each side is golden, about 3 minutes per side. Transfer to a baking dish.
3. In the same skillet, add the remaining olive oil, apples, and carrots. Sauté until

slightly softened, about 5 minutes. Sprinkle with cinnamon and black pepper.

4. Spread the sautéed apples and carrots over the chicken in the baking dish. Add the cooked grains around the chicken.

5. Pour vegetable broth over the ingredients in the baking dish. Cover with foil and bake for 20 minutes, or until the chicken is cooked through.

6. Serve hot, ensuring each plate gets an even mix of chicken, apples, carrots, and grains.

Nutritional Information (per serving):

- Calories: 320
- Protein: 28g
- Sodium: 180mg
- Potassium: 540mg
- Total Fat: 9g
- Saturated Fat: 1.5g
- Cholesterol: 75mg
- Carbohydrates: 35g
- Fiber: 5g

Chicken with Provencal Sauce

Prep Time: 15 minutes

Cooking Time: 30 minutes

Serving Size: 1 breast

Ingredients:

- 4 chicken breasts, boneless and skinless
- 1 tablespoon olive oil
- 1 onion, diced
- 2 cloves garlic, minced
- 1 can (14.5 ounces) no-salt-added diced tomatoes
- 1 teaspoon herbes de Provence
- Black pepper to taste
- 1/4 cup low-sodium chicken broth

Instructions:

1. Heat olive oil in a large skillet over medium heat. Add chicken breasts, cooking until golden on both sides, about 3 minutes per side. Remove chicken and set aside.

2. In the same skillet, add onion and garlic, cooking until softened, about 5 minutes.

3. Stir in diced tomatoes (with their juice), herbes de Provence, black pepper, and chicken broth. Bring to a simmer.

4. Return chicken to the skillet, covering it with the tomato mixture. Cover and simmer for 20 minutes, or until the chicken is cooked through.

5. Serve the chicken topped with the Provencal sauce.

Nutritional Information (per serving):

- Calories: 220
- Protein: 26g
- Sodium: 100mg
- Potassium: 600mg
- Total Fat: 8g
- Saturated Fat: 1.5g
- Cholesterol: 75mg
- Carbohydrates: 10g
- Fiber: 2g

Chicken with Quinoa and Wild Rice

Prep Time: 15 minutes

Cooking Time: 45 minutes

Serving Size: 1 portion

Ingredients:

- 1 cup quinoa, rinsed
- 1/2 cup wild rice
- 4 chicken breasts, boneless and skinless
- 2 tablespoons olive oil
- 1 onion, diced
- 2 cloves garlic, minced
- 2 cups low-sodium vegetable broth
- 1 teaspoon rosemary
- Black pepper to taste

Instructions:

1. In a medium saucepan, combine quinoa, wild rice, and 1 1/2 cups vegetable broth. Bring to a boil, then cover, reduce heat to low, and simmer for 45 minutes, or until grains are cooked and liquid is absorbed.
2. While grains are cooking, heat olive oil in a large skillet over medium heat. Add chicken breasts, seasoning with black pepper and rosemary. Cook until golden and cooked through, about 7 minutes per side. Remove and keep warm.
3. In the same skillet, add additional olive oil if needed, then cook onion and garlic until softened, about 5 minutes.
4. Slice the cooked chicken and serve over the cooked quinoa and wild rice mixture. Spoon the sautéed onions and garlic over the top.
5. Serve hot, accompanied by steamed vegetables if desired.

Nutritional Information (per serving):

- Calories: 330
- Protein: 29g
- Sodium: 150mg
- Potassium: 500mg
- Total Fat: 9g
- Saturated Fat: 1.5g
- Cholesterol: 65mg
- Carbohydrates: 35g
- Fiber: 5g

Easy Chicken and Pasta Dinner

Prep Time: 15 minutes

Cooking Time: 20 minutes

Serving Size: 1 cup

Ingredients:

- 2 chicken breasts, boneless and skinless
- 1 tablespoon olive oil
- 1 cup whole wheat pasta, uncooked
- 1 cup low-sodium chicken broth
- 1 cup spinach, fresh
- 1/2 cup cherry tomatoes, halved
- 1 garlic clove, minced
- Black pepper to taste
- 1 teaspoon oregano

1. Cook pasta according to package instructions, omitting salt. Drain and set aside.

2. In a skillet, heat olive oil over medium heat. Add chicken breasts and cook until golden brown on both sides and no longer pink in the middle, about 6-8 minutes per side. Remove chicken from skillet and set aside.

3. In the same skillet, add garlic and sauté for 1 minute. Add spinach and cherry tomatoes, cooking until spinach is wilted.

4. Slice the chicken into strips and return to the skillet. Add cooked pasta, low-sodium chicken broth, oregano, and black pepper. Toss everything together and cook for an additional 2-3 minutes.

5. Serve warm.

Nutritional Information (per serving):

- Calories: 320
- Protein: 28g
- Sodium: 100mg
- Potassium: 450mg
- Total Fat: 8g
- Saturated Fat: 1.5g
- Cholesterol: 65mg
- Carbohydrates: 35g
- Fiber: 6g

Easy Chicken Breasts in Herb Sauce for Two

Prep Time: 10 minutes

Cooking Time: 15 minutes

Serving Size: 1 breast

Ingredients:

- 2 chicken breasts, boneless and skinless
- 1 tablespoon olive oil
- 1/2 cup low-sodium chicken broth
- 1 teaspoon rosemary, minced
- 1 teaspoon thyme, minced
- 1 garlic clove, minced
- Black pepper to taste

Instructions:

1. Heat olive oil in a skillet over medium heat. Season chicken breasts with black pepper and add to the skillet. Cook until golden brown on each side, about 5-7 minutes per side.

2. Remove chicken breasts and set aside. In the same skillet, add garlic, rosemary, thyme, and low-sodium chicken broth. Bring to a simmer.

3. Return the chicken to the skillet, cover, and simmer for 5 minutes, or until the chicken is cooked through.

4. Serve the chicken breasts with the herb sauce spooned over the top.

Nutritional Information (per serving):

- Calories: 220
- Protein: 26g
- Sodium: 70mg

- Potassium: 370mg
- Total Fat: 10g
- Saturated Fat: 1.5g
- Cholesterol: 75mg
- Carbohydrates: 2g
- Fiber: 0.5g

Easy Chicken Enchiladas

Prep Time: 20 minutes

Cooking Time: 25 minutes

Serving Size: 2 enchiladas

Ingredients:

- 2 cups cooked chicken, shredded
- 1 cup low-sodium black beans, rinsed and drained
- 1 cup spinach, chopped
- 4 whole wheat tortillas
- 1 cup low-sodium enchilada sauce
- 1/2 cup shredded low-fat cheese
- 1 teaspoon cumin
- Black pepper to taste

Instructions:

1. Preheat oven to 375°F.
2. In a bowl, mix together shredded chicken, black beans, spinach, cumin, and black pepper.
3. Spoon the chicken mixture evenly onto each tortilla. Roll up and place seam-side down in a baking dish.
4. Pour enchilada sauce over the rolled tortillas and sprinkle with shredded cheese.
5. Cover with foil and bake for 20 minutes. Remove foil and bake for an additional 5 minutes, or until cheese is melted and bubbly.
6. Serve warm.

Nutritional Information (per serving):

- Calories: 350
- Protein: 28g
- Sodium: 200mg
- Potassium: 500mg
- Total Fat: 9g
- Saturated Fat: 2g
- Cholesterol: 60mg
- Carbohydrates: 35g
- Fiber: 6g

Easy Crispy Lemon Chicken

Prep Time: 10 minutes

Cooking Time: 20 minutes

Serving Size: 1 breast

Ingredients:

- 4 chicken breasts, boneless and skinless
- 1 tablespoon olive oil
- Juice and zest of 1 lemon
- 1 teaspoon paprika
- 1 garlic clove, minced
- Black pepper to taste

Instructions:

1. Preheat oven to 400°F.
2. In a bowl, combine lemon juice and zest, olive oil, paprika, garlic, and black pepper.

3. Place chicken breasts in a baking dish and pour the lemon mixture over them.

4. Bake for 20 minutes, or until the chicken is cooked through and the surface is crispy.

5. Serve warm, spooning any extra sauce from the baking dish over the chicken.

Nutritional Information (per serving):

- Calories: 220
- Protein: 26g
- Sodium: 70mg
- Potassium: 370mg
- Total Fat: 10g
- Saturated Fat: 1.5g
- Cholesterol: 75mg
- Carbohydrates: 3g
- Fiber: 0.5g

Garlic Chicken with Balsamic Vinegar

Prep Time: 10 minutes

Cooking Time: 20 minutes

Serving Size: 1 breast

Ingredients:

- 4 chicken breasts, boneless and skinless
- 2 tablespoons olive oil
- 4 garlic cloves, minced
- 1/4 cup balsamic vinegar
- 1 teaspoon thyme
- Black pepper to taste

Instructions:

1. Heat olive oil in a skillet over medium heat. Add the chicken breasts and cook until golden brown on each side, about 5-7 minutes per side. Remove chicken and set aside.

2. In the same skillet, add garlic and sauté for 1 minute. Add balsamic vinegar and thyme. Bring to a simmer.

3. Return the chicken to the skillet, cover, and simmer for 10 minutes, or until the chicken is cooked through.

4. Serve the chicken with the balsamic garlic sauce spooned over the top.

Nutritional Information (per serving):

- Calories: 230
- Protein: 27g
- Sodium: 75mg
- Potassium: 400mg
- Total Fat: 11g
- Saturated Fat: 1.5g
- Cholesterol: 75mg
- Carbohydrates: 4g
- Fiber: 0.5g

Glazed Cornish Game Hen for Two

Prep Time: 15 minutes

Cooking Time: 1 hour

Serving Size: 1/2 hen

Ingredients:

- 1 Cornish game hen, approximately 1.5 pounds, split in half
- 2 tablespoons olive oil
- 2 tablespoons balsamic vinegar
- 1 teaspoon rosemary, minced

* 1 teaspoon thyme, minced
* 2 cloves garlic, minced
* Black pepper to taste

Instructions:

1. Preheat oven to 375°F.
2. In a small bowl, mix olive oil, balsamic vinegar, rosemary, thyme, garlic, and black pepper to create the glaze.
3. Place the Cornish hen halves in a roasting pan. Brush them generously with the glaze.
4. Roast in the oven for about 1 hour, or until the internal temperature reaches 165°F, basting occasionally with the glaze.
5. Serve warm, garnished with additional herbs if desired.

Nutritional Information (per serving):

* Calories: 310
* Protein: 24g
* Sodium: 120mg
* Potassium: 370mg
* Total Fat: 22g
* Saturated Fat: 5g
* Cholesterol: 85mg
* Carbohydrates: 3g
* Fiber: 0g

Grilled Buttermilk Garlic Marinated Chicken

Prep Time: 4 hours (including marinating time)

Cooking Time: 20 minutes

Serving Size: 1 breast

Ingredients:

* 4 chicken breasts, boneless and skinless
* 1 cup low-fat buttermilk
* 4 cloves garlic, minced
* 1 tablespoon olive oil
* 1 teaspoon paprika
* Black pepper to taste

Instructions:

1. In a mixing bowl, combine buttermilk, garlic, olive oil, paprika, and black pepper.
2. Add chicken breasts to the mixture, ensuring they are fully coated. Cover and refrigerate for at least 4 hours, or overnight for best flavor.
3. Preheat grill to medium-high heat.
4. Remove chicken from marinade, discarding excess marinade. Grill chicken for about 10 minutes per side, or until fully cooked and internal temperature reaches 165°F.
5. Serve hot with your choice of side vegetables.

Nutritional Information (per serving):

* Calories: 260
* Protein: 31g

- Sodium: 150mg
- Potassium: 450mg
- Total Fat: 9g
- Saturated Fat: 2g
- Cholesterol: 80mg
- Carbohydrates: 5g
- Fiber: 0g

Grilled Chicken, Asparagus, and Corn

Prep Time: 15 minutes

Cooking Time: 20 minutes

Serving Size: 1 serving

Ingredients:

- 2 chicken breasts, boneless and skinless
- 1 bunch asparagus, ends trimmed
- 2 ears of corn, husks and silk removed
- 2 tablespoons olive oil
- Black pepper to taste
- 1 lemon, quartered, for serving

Instructions:

1. Preheat the grill to medium-high heat.
2. Brush the chicken, asparagus, and corn lightly with olive oil. Season with black pepper.
3. Grill chicken for about 6-7 minutes per side or until fully cooked. Grill asparagus and corn, turning occasionally, until tender and slightly charred, about 10 minutes.
4. Serve the grilled chicken, asparagus, and corn with lemon wedges on the side.

Nutritional Information (per serving):

- Calories: 320
- Protein: 28g
- Sodium: 90mg
- Potassium: 700mg
- Total Fat: 14g
- Saturated Fat: 2g
- Cholesterol: 70mg
- Carbohydrates: 22g
- Fiber: 4g

Homemade Chicken and Dumplings (or Turkey)

Prep Time: 30 minutes

Cooking Time: 1 hour

Serving Size: 1 bowl

Ingredients:

- 2 cups cooked chicken or turkey, shredded
- 6 cups low-sodium chicken or turkey broth
- 1 cup carrots, diced
- 1 cup celery, diced
- 1/2 cup onion, diced
- 1 cup all-purpose flour
- 2 teaspoons baking powder
- 1/2 cup low-fat milk
- 1 teaspoon thyme
- Black pepper to taste

Instructions:

1. In a large pot, bring the broth to a simmer. Add carrots, celery, onion, thyme, and black pepper. Cook until vegetables are tender, about 15 minutes.

2. In a bowl, mix flour, baking powder, and a pinch of black pepper. Stir in milk to form a dough.

3. Drop tablespoon-sized pieces of dough into the simmering broth. Cover and cook for about 15 minutes, or until dumplings are firm.

4. Add the cooked chicken or turkey to the pot and heat through.

5. Serve hot, ensuring each bowl gets an even mix of chicken (or turkey), vegetables, and dumplings.

Nutritional Information (per serving):

- Calories: 270
- Protein: 20g
- Sodium: 200mg
- Potassium: 400mg
- Total Fat: 6g
- Saturated Fat: 1.5g
- Cholesterol: 45mg
- Carbohydrates: 30g
- Fiber: 3g

Honey Mustard Grilled Chicken

Prep Time: 10 minutes (plus marinating time)

Cooking Time: 20 minutes

Serving Size: 1 breast

Ingredients:

- 4 chicken breasts, boneless and skinless
- 1/4 cup honey
- 1/4 cup Dijon mustard
- 2 tablespoons olive oil
- 1 tablespoon lemon juice
- 1 garlic clove, minced
- Black pepper to taste

Instructions:

1. In a bowl, whisk together honey, Dijon mustard, olive oil, lemon juice, garlic, and black pepper.

2. Place chicken breasts in a resealable plastic bag and pour the marinade over them. Ensure all pieces are coated. Marinate in the refrigerator for at least 1 hour, or overnight.

3. Preheat grill to medium-high heat.

4. Remove chicken from marinade, discarding any excess marinade. Grill for about 10 minutes per side, or until fully cooked and internal temperature reaches 165°F.

5. Serve hot, garnished with lemon slices or fresh herbs if desired.

Nutritional Information (per serving):

- Calories: 310
- Protein: 31g
- Sodium: 280mg
- Potassium: 450mg
- Total Fat: 12g
- Saturated Fat: 2g
- Cholesterol: 80mg
- Carbohydrates: 18g
- Fiber: 0g

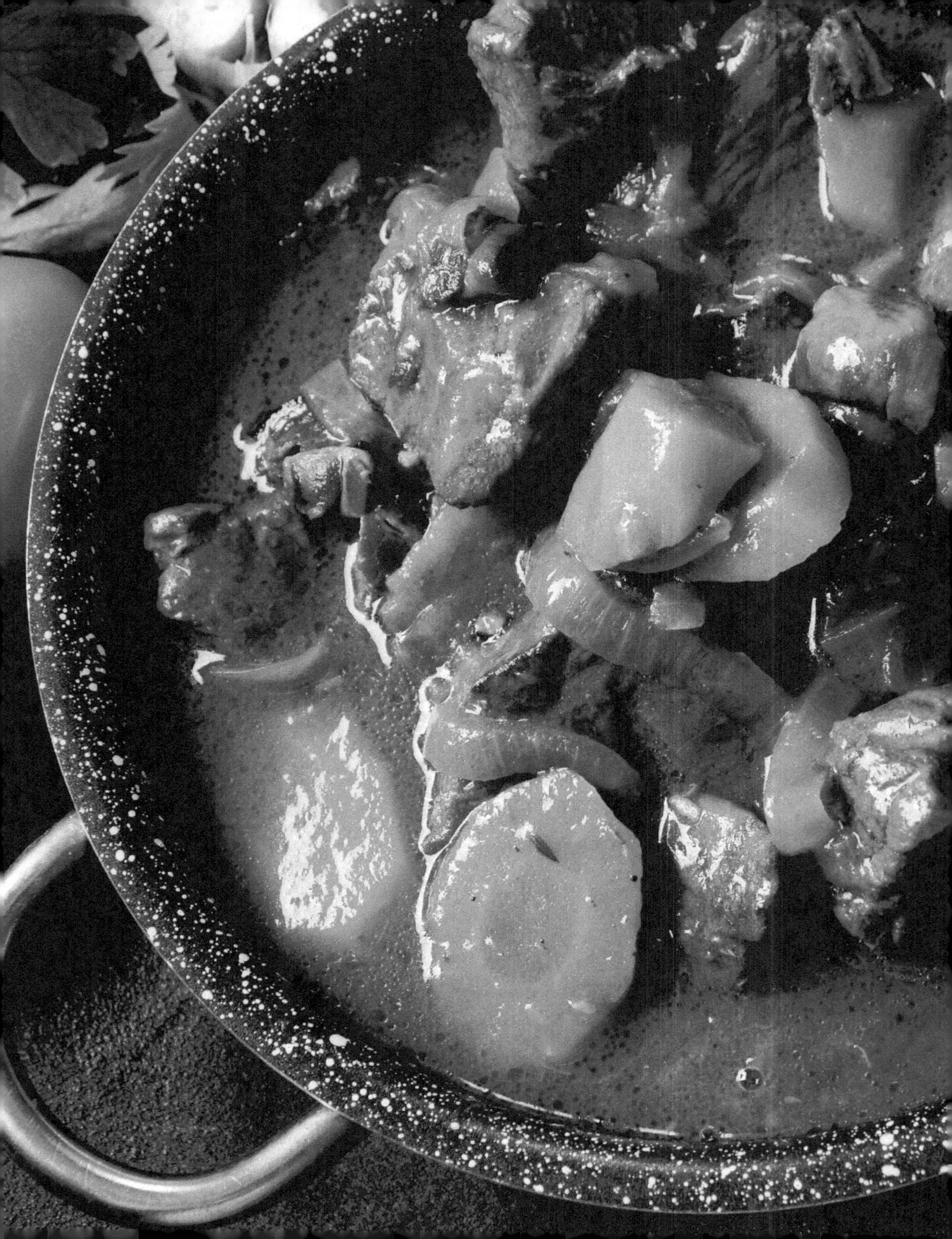

BEEF AND LAMB

Asian Lettuce Wraps

Prep Time: 20 minutes

Cooking Time: 10 minutes

Serving Size: 2 wraps

Ingredients:

- 1 pound ground turkey breast
- 1 tablespoon olive oil
- 1 cup mushrooms, finely chopped
- 1/2 cup carrots, shredded
- 1/4 cup green onions, chopped
- 2 garlic cloves, minced
- 1 tablespoon low-sodium soy sauce
- 1 teaspoon ginger, grated
- 1 tablespoon hoisin sauce
- 1 head of iceberg lettuce, leaves separated
- Fresh cilantro for garnish (optional)

Instructions:

1. Heat olive oil in a large skillet over medium heat. Add ground turkey and cook until browned, breaking it apart with a spoon.
2. Add mushrooms, carrots, green onions, and garlic to the skillet. Cook for another 5 minutes until the vegetables are soft.
3. Stir in low-sodium soy sauce, ginger, and hoisin sauce. Cook for an additional 2 minutes, stirring frequently.
4. Spoon the turkey mixture into the center of lettuce leaves. Garnish with fresh cilantro if desired.
5. Serve immediately as wraps.

Nutritional Information (per serving):

- Calories: 250
- Protein: 28g
- Sodium: 200mg
- Potassium: 650mg
- Total Fat: 8g
- Saturated Fat: 1g
- Cholesterol: 60mg
- Carbohydrates: 12g
- Fiber: 3g

Beef Burgundy Crepes

Prep Time: 30 minutes

Cooking Time: 2 hours

Serving Size: 2 crepes

Ingredients:

- 1/2 pound lean beef stew meat, cut into small pieces
- 1 tablespoon olive oil
- 1/4 cup onions, chopped
- 1/2 cup low-sodium beef broth
- 1/4 cup red wine (optional, can be replaced with additional beef broth)
- 1/2 cup mushrooms, sliced
- 1 teaspoon thyme
- Black pepper to taste

- 4 whole wheat crepes (prepared separately)
- Fresh parsley for garnish

Instructions:

1. In a large skillet, heat olive oil over medium heat. Add beef and onions, cooking until the beef is browned.
2. Add beef broth, red wine (if using), mushrooms, thyme, and black pepper. Bring to a boil, then reduce heat to low. Cover and simmer for about 1.5 to 2 hours until the beef is tender.
3. Spoon the beef mixture into the center of each crepe. Fold the crepes and serve garnished with fresh parsley.

Nutritional Information (per serving):

- Calories: 320
- Protein: 24g
- Sodium: 150mg
- Potassium: 500mg
- Total Fat: 12g
- Saturated Fat: 3g
- Cholesterol: 70mg
- Carbohydrates: 25g
- Fiber: 3g

Chinese Hotdish (Casserole)

Prep Time: 20 minutes

Cooking Time: 45 minutes

Serving Size: 1 cup

Ingredients:

- 1 pound ground turkey breast
- 1 tablespoon olive oil
- 1 cup celery, chopped
- 1/2 cup onions, chopped
- 1 cup cooked brown rice
- 1 cup low-sodium chicken broth
- 1/4 cup low-sodium soy sauce
- 1 cup frozen peas
- 1 teaspoon garlic powder
- 1 teaspoon ginger, grated

Instructions:

1. Preheat the oven to 350°F.
2. In a skillet, heat olive oil over medium heat. Add ground turkey, celery, and onions. Cook until the turkey is browned and vegetables are softened.
3. Stir in cooked brown rice, chicken broth, soy sauce, peas, garlic powder, and ginger. Mix well.
4. Transfer the mixture to a baking dish. Cover with foil and bake for 30 minutes. Uncover and bake for an additional 15 minutes until the top is slightly crispy.
5. Serve hot.

Nutritional Information (per serving):

- Calories: 220
- Protein: 22g
- Sodium: 300mg

- Potassium: 400mg
- Total Fat: 6g
- Saturated Fat: 1g
- Cholesterol: 45mg
- Carbohydrates: 20g
- Fiber: 3g

Chipotle-Glazed Mini Meat Loaves

Prep Time: 20 minutes

Cooking Time: 30 minutes

Serving Size: 1 mini loaf

Ingredients:

- 1 pound lean ground beef
- 1/2 cup whole wheat breadcrumbs
- 1 egg, beaten
- 1/4 cup low-sodium tomato sauce
- 1 chipotle pepper in adobo sauce, minced (adjust to taste)
- 1 teaspoon garlic powder
- 1 teaspoon onion powder
- Black pepper to taste

Instructions:

1. Preheat oven to 375°F.
2. In a bowl, combine ground beef, breadcrumbs, egg, 2 tablespoons of tomato sauce, chipotle pepper, garlic powder, onion powder, and black pepper.
3. Shape the mixture into 4 mini loaves and place on a baking sheet.
4. Mix the remaining tomato sauce with a bit of adobo sauce from the chipotle peppers. Brush this glaze over the mini meatloaves.
5. Bake for 30 minutes, or until the meatloaves reach an internal temperature of 160°F.
6. Serve hot.

Nutritional Information (per serving):

- Calories: 280
- Protein: 26g
- Sodium: 200mg
- Potassium: 450mg
- Total Fat: 12g
- Saturated Fat: 4g
- Cholesterol: 100mg
- Carbohydrates: 15g
- Fiber: 2g

Cream Cheesy Burgers

Prep Time: 15 minutes

Cooking Time: 10 minutes

Serving Size: 1 burger

Ingredients:

- 1 pound lean ground beef
- 2 ounces low-fat cream cheese, softened
- 1 tablespoon chives, chopped
- 1 teaspoon garlic powder
- Black pepper to taste
- 4 whole wheat burger buns
- Lettuce, tomato, and onion for serving

Instructions:

1. In a bowl, mix together ground beef, cream cheese, chives, garlic powder, and black pepper.

2. Form the mixture into 4 patties.

3. Grill or pan-fry the patties over medium heat for about 5 minutes per side, or until they reach the desired doneness.

4. Serve the burgers on whole wheat buns, topped with lettuce, tomato, and onion slices.

Nutritional Information (per serving):

- Calories: 350
- Protein: 28g
- Sodium: 250mg
- Potassium: 500mg
- Total Fat: 16g
- Saturated Fat: 6g
- Cholesterol: 80mg
- Carbohydrates: 25g
- Fiber: 4g

Easy BBQ Beef

Prep Time: 10 minutes

Cooking Time: 2 hours

Serving Size: 4 ounces

Ingredients:

- 2 pounds beef brisket, trimmed of excess fat
- 1 cup low-sodium beef broth
- 1/2 cup apple cider vinegar
- 2 tablespoons tomato paste
- 1 tablespoon Worcestershire sauce
- 1 tablespoon smoked paprika
- 1 teaspoon garlic powder
- 1 teaspoon onion powder
- Black pepper to taste

Instructions:

1. Preheat oven to 300°F.

2. In a bowl, mix together beef broth, apple cider vinegar, tomato paste, Worcestershire sauce, smoked paprika, garlic powder, onion powder, and black pepper.

3. Place the beef brisket in a large roasting pan. Pour the mixture over the brisket, ensuring it's well-coated.

4. Cover the pan with aluminum foil and bake for about 2 hours, or until the beef is tender and easily shreds with a fork.

5. Remove from oven, let it rest for 10 minutes, then shred the beef. Serve with the sauce from the pan drizzled on top.

Nutritional Information (per serving):

- Calories: 240
- Protein: 32g
- Sodium: 150mg
- Potassium: 500mg
- Total Fat: 10g
- Saturated Fat: 3g
- Cholesterol: 90mg
- Carbohydrates: 5g
- Fiber: 1g

Ground Beef and Green Pea Stove-top Casserole

Prep Time: 15 minutes

Cooking Time: 30 minutes

Serving Size: 1 cup

Ingredients:

- 1 pound lean ground beef
- 1 tablespoon olive oil
- 1/2 cup onions, diced
- 1 clove garlic, minced
- 1 cup frozen green peas
- 2 cups low-sodium beef broth
- 1 cup carrots, diced
- 1 teaspoon thyme
- Black pepper to taste

Instructions:

1. Heat olive oil in a large skillet over medium heat. Add ground beef, onions, and garlic. Cook until beef is browned.
2. Add frozen peas, beef broth, diced carrots, thyme, and black pepper. Stir well.
3. Bring to a simmer, then reduce heat to low. Cover and cook for 20 minutes, or until the vegetables are tender and the liquid is mostly absorbed.
4. Serve hot, garnished with fresh herbs if desired.

Nutritional Information (per serving):

- Calories: 220
- Protein: 26g
- Sodium: 100mg
- Potassium: 450mg
- Total Fat: 8g
- Saturated Fat: 2g
- Cholesterol: 70mg
- Carbohydrates: 10g
- Fiber: 3g

Ground Beef and Veggie Foil Pack Dinner

Prep Time: 20 minutes

Cooking Time: 25 minutes

Serving Size: 1 pack

Ingredients:

- 1 pound lean ground beef, formed into 4 patties
- 2 cups zucchini, sliced
- 2 cups bell peppers, sliced
- 1 teaspoon olive oil
- Black pepper to taste
- 1 teaspoon garlic powder

Instructions:

1. Preheat the grill to medium-high heat.
2. Cut 4 large pieces of aluminum foil. Place a beef patty in the center of each piece.
3. Toss zucchini and bell peppers with olive oil, black pepper, and garlic powder. Divide the vegetables evenly among the foil packs, placing them around the patties.
4. Fold the foil over the contents to seal the packs.

5. Grill for about 25 minutes, flipping halfway through, or until the beef is cooked to your desired doneness and vegetables are tender.

6. Carefully open the packs and serve.

Nutritional Information (per serving):

- Calories: 250
- Protein: 28g
- Sodium: 80mg
- Potassium: 650mg
- Total Fat: 10g
- Saturated Fat: 3g
- Cholesterol: 75mg
- Carbohydrates: 10g
- Fiber: 3g

Slow Roasted Beef Pot Roast with Carrots and Turnips

Prep Time: 15 minutes

Cooking Time: 3 hours

Serving Size: 4 ounces beef with vegetables

Ingredients:

- 2 pounds beef chuck roast
- 1 tablespoon olive oil
- 2 cups low-sodium beef broth
- 1 cup carrots, sliced
- 1 cup turnips, cubed
- 1 teaspoon rosemary
- Black pepper to taste

Instructions:

1. Preheat oven to 275°F.

2. Heat olive oil in a large Dutch oven over medium-high heat. Add beef and sear on all sides until browned.

3. Add beef broth, carrots, turnips, rosemary, and black pepper. Bring to a simmer.

4. Cover and place in the oven. Roast for about 3 hours, or until the beef is very tender.

5. Remove from oven, let rest for 10 minutes, then slice the beef. Serve with the vegetables and broth.

Nutritional Information (per serving):

- Calories: 310
- Protein: 34g
- Sodium: 150mg
- Potassium: 800mg
- Total Fat: 16g
- Saturated Fat: 5g
- Cholesterol: 100mg
- Carbohydrates: 8g
- Fiber: 2g

Southern Style Stuffed Peppers

Prep Time: 20 minutes

Cooking Time: 1 hour

Serving Size: 1 pepper

Ingredients:

- 4 large bell peppers, tops removed and seeded
- 1 pound lean ground beef
- 1 tablespoon olive oil
- 1/2 cup onions, chopped

- 1 cup cooked brown rice
- 1 cup low-sodium tomato sauce
- 1 teaspoon paprika
- Black pepper to taste
- 1/2 cup low-fat shredded cheddar cheese

Instructions:

1. Preheat oven to 350°F.
2. Heat olive oil in a skillet over medium heat. Add ground beef and onions, cooking until beef is browned.
3. Stir in cooked brown rice, half of the tomato sauce, paprika, and black pepper.
4. Fill each bell pepper with the beef and rice mixture. Place in a baking dish.
5. Pour the remaining tomato sauce over the stuffed peppers.
6. Cover with foil and bake for 45 minutes. Uncover, sprinkle with cheese, and bake for an additional 15 minutes, or until cheese is melted.
7. Serve hot.

Nutritional Information (per serving):

- Calories: 290
- Protein: 26g
- Sodium: 200mg
- Potassium: 750mg
- Total Fat: 12g
- Saturated Fat: 4g
- Cholesterol: 70mg
- Carbohydrates: 20g
- Fiber: 4g

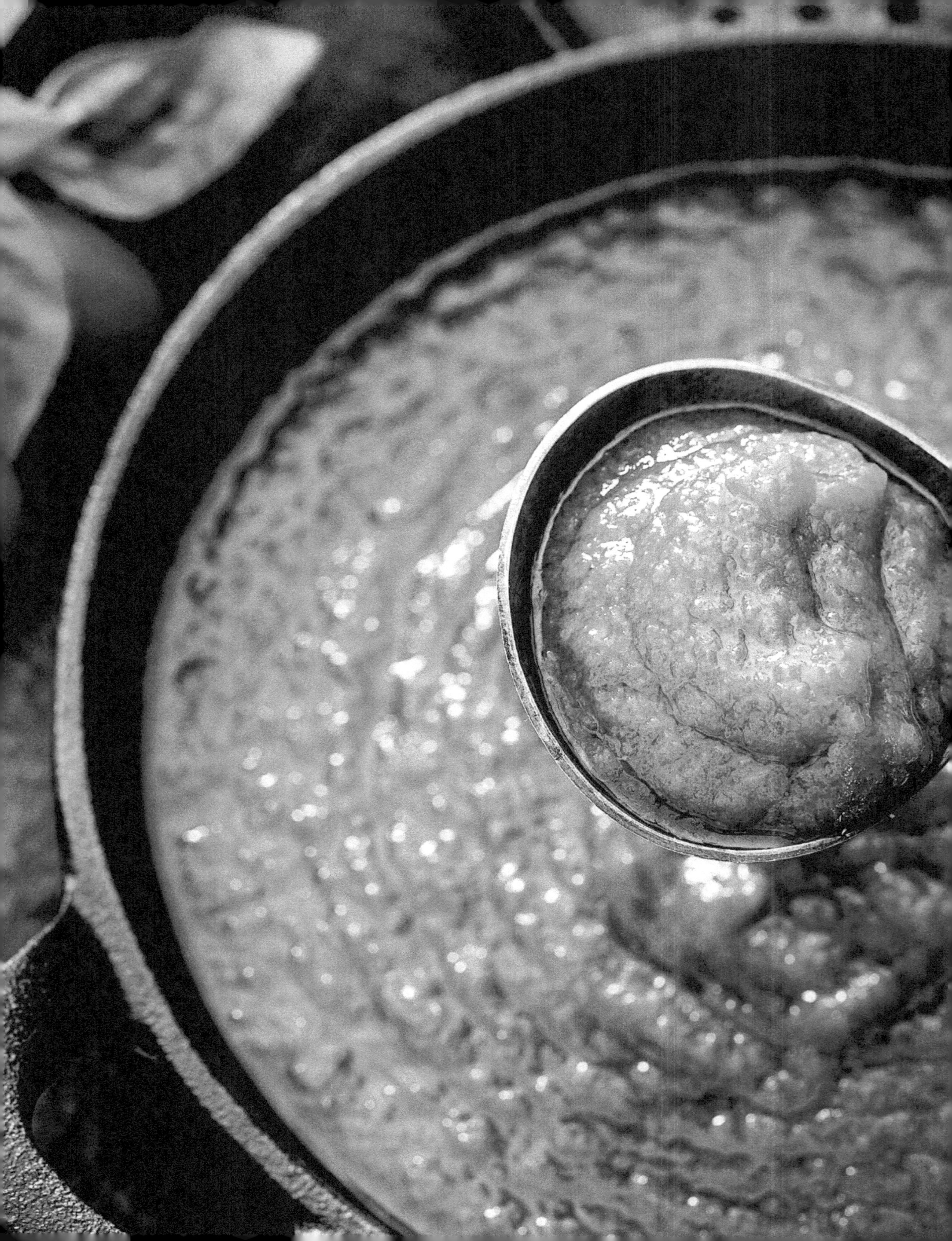

SAUCES & SEASONINGS

Adobo Seasoning

Prep Time: 5 minutes

Cooking Time: 0 minutes

Serving Size: 1/4 teaspoon

Ingredients:

- 2 tablespoons garlic powder
- 2 tablespoons onion powder
- 2 tablespoons dried oregano
- 1 tablespoon paprika
- 1 teaspoon ground black pepper
- 1 teaspoon ground turmeric

Instructions:

1. In a small bowl, combine all the ingredients thoroughly.
2. Store the adobo seasoning in an airtight container at room temperature.

Nutritional Information (per serving):

- Calories: 4
- Protein: 0.2g
- Sodium: 1mg
- Potassium: 10mg
- Total Fat: 0.1g
- Saturated Fat: 0g
- Cholesterol: 0mg
- Carbohydrates: 1g
- Fiber: 0.2g

Alfredo Sauce

Prep Time: 5 minutes

Cooking Time: 10 minutes

Serving Size: 1/4 cup

Ingredients:

- 1 cup low-fat milk
- 2 teaspoons olive oil
- 2 garlic cloves, minced
- 2 tablespoons all-purpose flour
- 1/2 cup grated Parmesan cheese, low sodium
- Black pepper to taste

Instructions:

1. Heat olive oil in a saucepan over medium heat. Add minced garlic and sauté until fragrant, about 1 minute.
2. Stir in flour to form a roux, cooking for another minute.
3. Gradually whisk in the milk, ensuring no lumps form. Cook until the sauce thickens, about 5 minutes.
4. Remove from heat and stir in grated Parmesan cheese until smooth. Season with black pepper.
5. Serve over cooked pasta or vegetables.

Nutritional Information (per serving):

- Calories: 60
- Protein: 4g
- Sodium: 90mg
- Potassium: 45mg

- Total Fat: 3.5g
- Saturated Fat: 1.5g
- Cholesterol: 5mg
- Carbohydrates: 4g
- Fiber: 0g

Basic Meat Coating Mix

Prep Time: 5 minutes

Cooking Time: 0 minutes

Serving Size: 1 tablespoon

Ingredients:

- 1 cup all-purpose flour
- 1 tablespoon garlic powder
- 1 tablespoon onion powder
- 1 teaspoon paprika
- 1 teaspoon ground black pepper

Instructions:

1. In a bowl, combine all the ingredients and mix well.
2. Store the coating mix in an airtight container. To use, coat pieces of meat evenly before cooking.

Nutritional Information (per serving):

- Calories: 28
- Protein: 0.8g
- Sodium: 2mg
- Potassium: 16mg
- Total Fat: 0.1g
- Saturated Fat: 0g
- Cholesterol: 0mg
- Carbohydrates: 6g
- Fiber: 0.4g

Basic White Sauce

Prep Time: 5 minutes

Cooking Time: 10 minutes

Serving Size: 1/4 cup

Ingredients:

- 2 tablespoons unsalted butter
- 2 tablespoons all-purpose flour
- 1 cup low-fat milk
- Black pepper to taste

Instructions:

1. Melt butter in a saucepan over medium heat. Stir in flour to form a smooth paste.
2. Gradually add milk, whisking constantly to prevent lumps. Cook until the sauce thickens, about 5 minutes.
3. Season with black pepper. Serve as a base for other sauces or as a topping for vegetables and pasta.

Nutritional Information (per serving):

- Calories: 45
- Protein: 1.5g
- Sodium: 25mg
- Potassium: 50mg
- Total Fat: 3g
- Saturated Fat: 1.8g
- Cholesterol: 8mg
- Carbohydrates: 3g
- Fiber: 0g

Basil Pesto

Prep Time: 10 minutes

Cooking Time: 0 minutes

Serving Size: 1 tablespoon

Ingredients:

- 2 cups fresh basil leaves
- 1/4 cup pine nuts
- 2 garlic cloves
- 1/2 cup grated Parmesan cheese, low sodium
- 1/4 cup olive oil
- Black pepper to taste

Instructions:

1. In a food processor, combine basil leaves, pine nuts, garlic, and Parmesan cheese. Pulse until coarsely chopped.
2. With the processor running, gradually add olive oil until well blended and smooth.
3. Season with black pepper. Store in an airtight container in the refrigerator.

Nutritional Information (per serving):

- Calories: 80
- Protein: 2g
- Sodium: 45mg
- Potassium: 25mg
- Total Fat: 8g
- Saturated Fat: 1.5g
- Cholesterol: 2mg
- Carbohydrates: 1g
- Fiber: 0.2g

Beef Brisket Gravy

Prep Time: 5 minutes

Cooking Time: Depends on brisket

Serving Size: 1/4 cup

Ingredients:

- Drippings from a cooked beef brisket
- 2 tablespoons all-purpose flour
- 1 cup low-sodium beef broth
- Black pepper to taste

Instructions:

1. After cooking the beef brisket, remove the meat and place the roasting pan over medium heat.
2. Stir in flour, mixing with the drippings to create a smooth paste.
3. Gradually whisk in beef broth, scraping up any browned bits from the bottom of the pan. Cook until the gravy thickens, about 5 minutes.
4. Season with black pepper. Strain the gravy through a fine mesh sieve before serving.

Nutritional Information (per serving):

- Calories: 30
- Protein: 1g
- Sodium: 45mg
- Potassium: 50mg
- Total Fat: 1.5g
- Saturated Fat: 0.5g
- Cholesterol: 5mg
- Carbohydrates: 3g
- Fiber: 0g

Blackberry Sauce

Prep Time: 5 minutes

Cooking Time: 10 minutes

Serving Size: 2 tablespoons

Ingredients:

- 2 cups fresh blackberries
- 1/4 cup water
- 2 tablespoons lemon juice
- 1 tablespoon honey (adjust based on taste and dietary restrictions)

Instructions:

1. In a saucepan over medium heat, combine blackberries, water, lemon juice, and honey.
2. Bring to a simmer, stirring occasionally, until the blackberries break down and the sauce thickens, about 10 minutes.
3. Use a fine mesh strainer to strain the sauce, discarding the seeds and pulp.
4. Allow the sauce to cool before serving. It can be used as a topping for desserts or meats.

Nutritional Information (per serving):

- Calories: 30
- Protein: 0.5g
- Sodium: 1mg
- Potassium: 70mg
- Total Fat: 0.2g
- Saturated Fat: 0g
- Cholesterol: 0mg
- Carbohydrates: 7g
- Fiber: 2g

Cucumber Dill Salsa

Prep Time: 10 minutes

Cooking Time: 0 minutes

Serving Size: 1/4 cup

Ingredients:

- 2 cups cucumber, diced
- 1/4 cup red onion, finely chopped
- 2 tablespoons fresh dill, chopped
- 2 tablespoons lemon juice
- 1 tablespoon olive oil
- Black pepper to taste

Instructions:

1. In a bowl, combine cucumber, red onion, fresh dill, lemon juice, and olive oil. Toss gently to mix.
2. Season with black pepper to taste.
3. Refrigerate for at least 30 minutes before serving to allow flavors to meld.
4. Serve as a refreshing side dish or with grilled meats and fish.

Nutritional Information (per serving):

- Calories: 25
- Protein: 0.5g
- Sodium: 2mg
- Potassium: 115mg
- Total Fat: 1.5g
- Saturated Fat: 0.2g
- Cholesterol: 0mg
- Carbohydrates: 3g
- Fiber: 0.5g

Curried Onion and Garlic Seasoning

Prep Time: 5 minutes

Cooking Time: 0 minutes

Serving Size: 1 teaspoon

Ingredients:

- 2 tablespoons onion powder
- 2 tablespoons garlic powder
- 1 tablespoon ground turmeric
- 1 tablespoon ground coriander
- 1 tablespoon ground cumin
- 1 teaspoon black pepper

Instructions:

1. In a small bowl, mix together onion powder, garlic powder, turmeric, coriander, cumin, and black pepper until well combined.
2. Store the seasoning blend in an airtight container in a cool, dry place.
3. Use as a seasoning for meats, vegetables, or any dish needing a flavor boost.

Nutritional Information (per serving):

- Calories: 8
- Protein: 0.4g
- Sodium: 2mg
- Potassium: 28mg
- Total Fat: 0.2g
- Saturated Fat: 0g
- Cholesterol: 0mg
- Carbohydrates: 1.5g
- Fiber: 0.5g

Garlic Sauce

Prep Time: 5 minutes

Cooking Time: 5 minutes

Serving Size: 2 tablespoons

Ingredients:

- 1/4 cup low-fat Greek yogurt
- 2 cloves garlic, minced
- 1 tablespoon lemon juice
- 1 teaspoon olive oil
- Black pepper to taste

Instructions:

1. In a bowl, whisk together Greek yogurt, minced garlic, lemon juice, and olive oil until smooth.
2. Season with black pepper to taste.
3. Refrigerate until ready to serve. This sauce is excellent with grilled meats, vegetables, or as a dip.

Nutritional Information (per serving):

- Calories: 25
- Protein: 1g
- Sodium: 10mg
- Potassium: 35mg
- Total Fat: 1.5g
- Saturated Fat: 0.2g
- Cholesterol: 1mg
- Carbohydrates: 2g
- Fiber: 0g

Grilled Pineapple Salsa

Prep Time: 15 minutes (plus grilling time)

Cooking Time: 10 minutes

Serving Size: 1/4 cup

Ingredients:

- 1 cup pineapple, sliced into rings
- 1/4 cup red bell pepper, diced
- 1/4 cup red onion, finely chopped
- 2 tablespoons cilantro, chopped
- 1 tablespoon lime juice
- Black pepper to taste

Instructions:

1. Preheat the grill to medium-high heat. Grill pineapple rings until charred, about 3-4 minutes per side.
2. Once cooled, dice the grilled pineapple and place it in a bowl.
3. Add red bell pepper, red onion, cilantro, and lime juice to the bowl with the pineapple. Toss to combine.
4. Season with black pepper to taste.
5. Serve as a topping for grilled meats or as a refreshing side dish.

Nutritional Information (per serving):

- Calories: 25
- Protein: 0.4g
- Sodium: 1mg
- Potassium: 85mg
- Total Fat: 0.1g
- Saturated Fat: 0g
- Cholesterol: 0mg
- Carbohydrates: 6g
- Fiber: 0.7g

Blackberry Sauce

Prep Time: 5 minutes

Cooking Time: 10 minutes

Serving Size: 2 tablespoons

Ingredients:

- 2 cups fresh blackberries
- 1/4 cup water
- 2 tablespoons lemon juice
- 1 tablespoon honey (adjust based on taste and dietary restrictions)

Instructions:

1. In a saucepan over medium heat, combine blackberries, water, lemon juice, and honey.
2. Bring to a simmer, stirring occasionally, until the blackberries break down and the sauce thickens, about 10 minutes.
3. Use a fine mesh strainer to strain the sauce, discarding the seeds and pulp.
4. Allow the sauce to cool before serving. It can be used as a topping for desserts or meats.

Nutritional Information (per serving):

- Calories: 30
- Protein: 0.5g
- Sodium: 1mg
- Potassium: 70mg
- Total Fat: 0.2g
- Saturated Fat: 0g
- Cholesterol: 0mg
- Carbohydrates: 7g
- Fiber: 2g

Cucumber Dill Salsa

Prep Time: 10 minutes

Cooking Time: 0 minutes

Serving Size: 1/4 cup

Ingredients:

- 2 cups cucumber, diced
- 1/4 cup red onion, finely chopped
- 2 tablespoons fresh dill, chopped
- 2 tablespoons lemon juice
- 1 tablespoon olive oil
- Black pepper to taste

Instructions:

1. In a bowl, combine cucumber, red onion, fresh dill, lemon juice, and olive oil. Toss gently to mix.
2. Season with black pepper to taste.
3. Refrigerate for at least 30 minutes before serving to allow flavors to meld.
4. Serve as a refreshing side dish or with grilled meats and fish.

Nutritional Information (per serving):

- Calories: 25
- Protein: 0.5g
- Sodium: 2mg
- Potassium: 115mg
- Total Fat: 1.5g
- Saturated Fat: 0.2g
- Cholesterol: 0mg
- Carbohydrates: 3g
- Fiber: 0.5g

Curried Onion and Garlic Seasoning

Prep Time: 5 minutes

Cooking Time: 0 minutes

Serving Size: 1 teaspoon

Ingredients:

- 2 tablespoons onion powder
- 2 tablespoons garlic powder
- 1 tablespoon ground turmeric
- 1 tablespoon ground coriander
- 1 tablespoon ground cumin
- 1 teaspoon black pepper

Instructions:

1. In a small bowl, mix together onion powder, garlic powder, turmeric, coriander, cumin, and black pepper until well combined.
2. Store the seasoning blend in an airtight container in a cool, dry place.
3. Use as a seasoning for meats, vegetables, or any dish needing a flavor boost.

Nutritional Information (per serving):

- Calories: 8
- Protein: 0.4g
- Sodium: 2mg
- Potassium: 28mg
- Total Fat: 0.2g
- Saturated Fat: 0g
- Cholesterol: 0mg
- Carbohydrates: 1.5g
- Fiber: 0.5g

Garlic Sauce

Prep Time: 5 minutes

Cooking Time: 5 minutes

Serving Size: 2 tablespoons

Ingredients:

- 1/4 cup low-fat Greek yogurt
- 2 cloves garlic, minced
- 1 tablespoon lemon juice
- 1 teaspoon olive oil
- Black pepper to taste

Instructions:

1. In a bowl, whisk together Greek yogurt, minced garlic, lemon juice, and olive oil until smooth.
2. Season with black pepper to taste.
3. Refrigerate until ready to serve. This sauce is excellent with grilled meats, vegetables, or as a dip.

Nutritional Information (per serving):

- Calories: 25
- Protein: 1g
- Sodium: 10mg
- Potassium: 35mg
- Total Fat: 1.5g
- Saturated Fat: 0.2g
- Cholesterol: 1mg
- Carbohydrates: 2g
- Fiber: 0g

Grilled Pineapple Salsa

Prep Time: 15 minutes (plus grilling time)

Cooking Time: 10 minutes

Serving Size: 1/4 cup

Ingredients:

- 1 cup pineapple, sliced into rings
- 1/4 cup red bell pepper, diced
- 1/4 cup red onion, finely chopped
- 2 tablespoons cilantro, chopped
- 1 tablespoon lime juice
- Black pepper to taste

Instructions:

1. Preheat the grill to medium-high heat. Grill pineapple rings until charred, about 3-4 minutes per side.
2. Once cooled, dice the grilled pineapple and place it in a bowl.
3. Add red bell pepper, red onion, cilantro, and lime juice to the bowl with the pineapple. Toss to combine.
4. Season with black pepper to taste.
5. Serve as a topping for grilled meats or as a refreshing side dish.

Nutritional Information (per serving):

- Calories: 25
- Protein: 0.4g
- Sodium: 1mg
- Potassium: 85mg
- Total Fat: 0.1g
- Saturated Fat: 0g
- Cholesterol: 0mg
- Carbohydrates: 6g
- Fiber: 0.7g

SOUPS & STEWS

Apple Cider Beef Stew

Prep Time: 20 minutes

Cooking Time: 2 hours

Serving Size: 1 cup

Ingredients:

- 1 pound lean beef stew meat, cut into cubes
- 1 tablespoon olive oil
- 2 cups low-sodium beef broth
- 1 cup apple cider (ensure low sugar content)
- 2 carrots, peeled and diced
- 2 parsnips, peeled and diced
- 1 onion, diced
- 2 cloves garlic, minced
- 1 teaspoon dried thyme
- 1 bay leaf
- Black pepper to taste

Instructions:

1. Heat olive oil in a large pot over medium-high heat. Add beef cubes and brown on all sides.
2. Add the low-sodium beef broth and apple cider to the pot. Bring to a simmer.
3. Add carrots, parsnips, onion, garlic, thyme, bay leaf, and black pepper. Stir well.
4. Reduce heat to low, cover, and simmer for about 2 hours, or until the beef is tender and the vegetables are cooked.
5. Remove the bay leaf before serving. Serve hot.

Nutritional Information (per serving):

- Calories: 220
- Protein: 25g
- Sodium: 150mg
- Potassium: 450mg
- Total Fat: 8g
- Saturated Fat: 2g
- Cholesterol: 60mg
- Carbohydrates: 15g
- Fiber: 3g

Asian Soup Jar

Prep Time: 10 minutes

Assembly Time: 5 minutes

Serving Size: 1 jar

Ingredients:

- 1/2 cup cooked, shredded chicken breast
- 1/4 cup rice noodles, cooked
- 1/4 cup shredded carrots
- 1/4 cup sliced mushrooms
- 1 tablespoon green onions, sliced
- 1 teaspoon low-sodium soy sauce
- 1/2 teaspoon ginger, grated
- 1 cup low-sodium chicken broth

Instructions:

1. In a heat-proof jar, layer the cooked chicken, rice noodles, shredded carrots, sliced mushrooms, and green onions.

2. In a small bowl, mix together the low-sodium soy sauce and grated ginger. Pour this mixture into the jar.

3. When ready to eat, pour hot low-sodium chicken broth into the jar to fill. Close the lid and let sit for 3-5 minutes.

4. Stir well before eating. Enjoy hot.

Nutritional Information (per serving):

- Calories: 180
- Protein: 18g
- Sodium: 200mg
- Potassium: 300mg
- Total Fat: 3g
- Saturated Fat: 0.5g
- Cholesterol: 40mg
- Carbohydrates: 20g
- Fiber: 2g

Cabbage Borscht

Prep Time: 20 minutes

Cooking Time: 1 hour

Serving Size: 1 cup

Ingredients:

- 1 pound lean beef, cut into cubes
- 1 tablespoon olive oil
- 4 cups shredded cabbage
- 2 beets, peeled and shredded
- 1 onion, diced
- 2 cloves garlic, minced
- 6 cups low-sodium beef broth
- 2 tablespoons tomato paste
- 1 tablespoon vinegar
- Black pepper to taste
- Fresh dill for garnish

Instructions:

1. In a large pot, heat olive oil over medium heat. Add beef and brown on all sides.

2. Add shredded cabbage, beets, onion, and garlic to the pot. Cook for 5 minutes, stirring occasionally.

3. Pour in the low-sodium beef broth. Stir in tomato paste and vinegar. Season with black pepper.

4. Bring to a boil, then reduce heat to low and simmer for about 1 hour, or until the beef is tender and the vegetables are cooked.

5. Garnish with fresh dill before serving. Serve hot.

Nutritional Information (per serving):

- Calories: 150
- Protein: 16g
- Sodium: 150mg
- Potassium: 500mg
- Total Fat: 5g
- Saturated Fat: 1.5g
- Cholesterol: 40mg
- Carbohydrates: 10g
- Fiber: 3g

Chicken Chili

Prep Time: 15 minutes

Cooking Time: 30 minutes

Serving Size: 1 cup

Ingredients:

- 1 pound ground chicken breast
- 1 tablespoon olive oil
- 1 onion, diced
- 2 cloves garlic, minced
- 1 can (15 ounces) low-sodium white beans, drained and rinsed
- 1 can (15 ounces) low-sodium diced tomatoes
- 1 cup low-sodium chicken broth
- 1 teaspoon ground cumin
- 1 teaspoon paprika
- Black pepper to taste
- Fresh cilantro for garnish

Instructions:

1. Heat olive oil in a large pot over medium heat. Add ground chicken, onion, and garlic. Cook until the chicken is no longer pink.
2. Stir in white beans, diced tomatoes, chicken broth, cumin, paprika, and black pepper.
3. Bring to a simmer and cook for 25-30 minutes, stirring occasionally.
4. Garnish with fresh cilantro before serving. Serve hot.

Nutritional Information (per serving):

- Calories: 210
- Protein: 22g
- Sodium: 200mg
- Potassium: 600mg
- Total Fat: 6g
- Saturated Fat: 1g
- Cholesterol: 55mg
- Carbohydrates: 18g
- Fiber: 5g

Chicken Corn Soup

Prep Time: 10 minutes

Cooking Time: 20 minutes

Serving Size: 1 cup

Ingredients:

- 1/2 pound cooked chicken breast, shredded
- 1 tablespoon olive oil
- 1 onion, diced
- 2 cloves garlic, minced
- 1 cup frozen corn
- 4 cups low-sodium chicken broth
- 1/4 cup fresh parsley, chopped
- Black pepper to taste

Instructions:

1. Heat olive oil in a large pot over medium heat. Add onion and garlic, sautéing until translucent.
2. Add frozen corn and cooked shredded chicken to the pot. Stir to combine.
3. Pour in low-sodium chicken broth and bring to a simmer.
4. Simmer for 15 minutes, allowing flavors to meld.

5. Stir in fresh parsley and season with black pepper to taste before serving. Serve hot.

Nutritional Information (per serving):

- Calories: 120
- Protein: 14g
- Sodium: 150mg
- Potassium: 300mg
- Total Fat: 3.5g
- Saturated Fat: 0.5g
- Cholesterol: 30mg
- Carbohydrates: 8g
- Fiber: 1g

Chicken Noodle Soup

Prep Time: 15 minutes

Cooking Time: 30 minutes

Serving Size: 1 cup

Ingredients:

- 1/2 pound chicken breast, cubed
- 1 tablespoon olive oil
- 4 cups low-sodium chicken broth
- 1 cup carrots, sliced
- 1/2 cup celery, sliced
- 1/2 cup onion, diced
- 2 cloves garlic, minced
- 1/2 cup whole wheat noodles
- 1 teaspoon thyme
- Black pepper to taste
- 2 tablespoons fresh parsley, chopped

Instructions:

1. In a large pot, heat olive oil over medium heat. Add chicken and cook until no longer pink.
2. Add carrots, celery, onion, and garlic. Sauté until vegetables are softened, about 5 minutes.
3. Pour in low-sodium chicken broth and bring to a boil.
4. Add whole wheat noodles, thyme, and black pepper. Reduce heat and simmer for 20 minutes, or until noodles are tender.
5. Stir in fresh parsley before serving. Serve hot.

Nutritional Information (per serving):

- Calories: 120
- Protein: 14g
- Sodium: 100mg
- Potassium: 200mg
- Total Fat: 3g
- Saturated Fat: 0.5g
- Cholesterol: 30mg
- Carbohydrates: 10g
- Fiber: 2g

Chicken Wild Rice Soup

Prep Time: 20 minutes

Cooking Time: 1 hour

Serving Size: 1 cup

Ingredients:

- 1/2 pound chicken breast, cubed
- 1 tablespoon olive oil
- 4 cups low-sodium chicken broth
- 1 cup wild rice, rinsed
- 1 cup mushrooms, sliced
- 1/2 cup carrots, diced
- 1/2 cup celery, diced
- 1 onion, diced
- 1 clove garlic, minced
- 1 teaspoon thyme
- Black pepper to taste

Instructions:

1. In a large pot, heat olive oil over medium heat. Add chicken and cook until browned.
2. Add mushrooms, carrots, celery, onion, and garlic. Cook until vegetables are softened, about 10 minutes.
3. Stir in low-sodium chicken broth, wild rice, thyme, and black pepper. Bring to a boil.
4. Reduce heat, cover, and simmer for about 45 minutes, or until the rice is tender.
5. Adjust seasoning if necessary. Serve hot, garnished with fresh herbs if desired.

Nutritional Information (per serving):

- Calories: 130
- Protein: 15g
- Sodium: 100mg
- Potassium: 250mg
- Total Fat: 3g
- Saturated Fat: 0.5g
- Cholesterol: 30mg
- Carbohydrates: 14g
- Fiber: 2g

Moroccan Chicken Soup

Prep Time: 20 minutes

Cooking Time: 40 minutes

Serving Size: 1 cup

Ingredients:

- 1/2 pound chicken breast, cubed
- 1 tablespoon olive oil
- 4 cups low-sodium chicken broth
- 1 cup diced tomatoes, no salt added
- 1/2 cup lentils, rinsed
- 1 carrot, diced
- 1 celery stalk, diced
- 1 onion, diced
- 2 cloves garlic, minced
- 1 teaspoon cumin
- 1 teaspoon paprika
- 1/2 teaspoon cinnamon
- Black pepper to taste
- 2 tablespoons cilantro, chopped

Instructions:

1. In a large pot, heat olive oil over medium heat. Add chicken and cook until no longer pink.

2. Add carrots, celery, onion, and garlic. Cook until vegetables are softened, about 10 minutes.

3. Stir in low-sodium chicken broth, diced tomatoes, lentils, cumin, paprika, cinnamon, and black pepper. Bring to a boil.

4. Reduce heat and simmer for 30 minutes, or until lentils are tender.

5. Garnish with cilantro before serving. Serve hot.

Nutritional Information (per serving):

- Calories: 150
- Protein: 16g
- Sodium: 100mg
- Potassium: 300mg
- Total Fat: 3g
- Saturated Fat: 0.5g

BEVERAGES

Almond Vanilla Espresso

Prep Time: 5 minutes

Cooking Time: 0 minutes

Serving Size: 1 cup

Ingredients:

- 1 cup brewed espresso, cooled
- 1/2 cup unsweetened almond milk
- 1 teaspoon vanilla extract
- Ice cubes
- 1 tablespoon almond syrup (sugar-free if necessary)

Instructions:

1. In a large cup, mix the cooled espresso with vanilla extract and almond syrup.
2. Fill a glass with ice cubes to the top.
3. Pour the almond milk into the glass, then add the espresso mixture.
4. Stir well to combine all the ingredients. Serve immediately.

Nutritional Information (per serving):

- Calories: 30
- Protein: 1g
- Sodium: 50mg
- Potassium: 75mg
- Total Fat: 2g
- Saturated Fat: 0g
- Cholesterol: 0mg
- Carbohydrates: 3g
- Fiber: 0.5g

Champagne Punch

Prep Time: 10 minutes

Cooking Time: 0 minutes

Serving Size: 1 cup

Ingredients:

- 1 bottle low-sugar sparkling white grape juice, chilled
- 1 cup unsweetened cranberry juice, chilled
- 1 liter sparkling water, chilled
- 1 cup mixed fresh fruit (strawberries, blueberries, raspberries)
- Ice cubes

Instructions:

1. In a large punch bowl, combine sparkling white grape juice, cranberry juice, and sparkling water.
2. Add fresh fruit to the mixture.
3. Add ice cubes just before serving to keep the punch chilled without diluting it too much.
4. Serve in punch cups or glasses.

Nutritional Information (per serving):

- Calories: 50
- Protein: 0g
- Sodium: 10mg
- Potassium: 120mg
- Total Fat: 0g
- Saturated Fat: 0g
- Cholesterol: 0mg

- Carbohydrates: 12g
- Fiber: 1g

Chocolate Smoothie

Prep Time: 5 minutes

Cooking Time: 0 minutes

Serving Size: 1 cup

Ingredients:

- 1 cup unsweetened almond milk
- 1 banana, frozen
- 1 tablespoon unsweetened cocoa powder
- 1/2 teaspoon vanilla extract
- 1 tablespoon chia seeds
- Ice cubes

Instructions:

1. Place almond milk, frozen banana, cocoa powder, vanilla extract, and chia seeds into a blender.
2. Blend on high until smooth.
3. Add ice cubes and blend again until the desired consistency is reached.
4. Serve immediately in a chilled glass.

Nutritional Information (per serving):

- Calories: 150
- Protein: 3g
- Sodium: 90mg
- Potassium: 400mg
- Total Fat: 4g
- Saturated Fat: 0.5g
- Cholesterol: 0mg
- Carbohydrates: 27g
- Fiber: 6g

High Protein Piña Colada

Prep Time: 5 minutes

Cooking Time: 0 minutes

Serving Size: 1 cup

Ingredients:

- 1 cup frozen pineapple chunks
- 1/2 cup canned coconut milk, light
- 1/2 cup unsweetened almond milk
- 1 scoop vanilla whey protein powder (low in potassium and phosphorus)
- Ice cubes

Instructions:

1. Place pineapple chunks, coconut milk, almond milk, and protein powder into a blender.
2. Blend on high until smooth.
3. Add ice cubes and blend again until the desired consistency is reached.
4. Serve immediately in a chilled glass.

Nutritional Information (per serving):

- Calories: 200
- Protein: 15g
- Sodium: 50mg
- Potassium: 200mg
- Total Fat: 8g
- Saturated Fat: 5g
- Cholesterol: 30mg
- Carbohydrates: 18g
- Fiber: 2g

High Protein Rice Milk

Prep Time: 5 minutes plus soaking time

Cooking Time: 0 minutes

Serving Size: 1 cup

Ingredients:

- 1 cup cooked brown rice
- 4 cups water
- 1 scoop vanilla whey protein powder (low in potassium and phosphorus)
- 1 teaspoon vanilla extract
- 1 tablespoon honey (optional)

Instructions:

1. Soak cooked brown rice in water for at least 2 hours or overnight in the refrigerator.
2. Blend soaked rice and water until smooth.
3. Strain the mixture using a nut milk bag or fine mesh sieve to remove the solid parts.
4. Return the liquid to the blender, add protein powder, vanilla extract, and honey (if using), and blend until smooth.
5. Serve chilled. Store any leftovers in a sealed container in the refrigerator.

Nutritional Information (per serving):

- Calories: 100
- Protein: 8g
- Sodium: 40mg
- Potassium: 70mg
- Total Fat: 1g
- Saturated Fat: 0.5g
- Cholesterol: 15mg
- Carbohydrates: 14g
- Fiber: 1g

Homemade Rice Milk

Prep Time: 5 minutes plus soaking time

Cooking Time: 0 minutes

Serving Size: 1 cup

Ingredients:

- 1 cup cooked brown rice
- 4 cups water
- 1 teaspoon vanilla extract
- 1 tablespoon honey (optional)

Instructions:

1. Soak cooked brown rice in water for at least 2 hours or overnight in the refrigerator.
2. Blend soaked rice and water until smooth.
3. Strain the mixture using a nut milk bag or fine mesh sieve to remove the solid parts.
4. Stir in vanilla extract and honey (if using) until well combined.
5. Serve chilled. Store any leftovers in a sealed container in the refrigerator.

Nutritional Information (per serving):

- Calories: 70
- Protein: 1g
- Sodium: 10mg
- Potassium: 40mg
- Total Fat: 0.5g
- Saturated Fat: 0g
- Cholesterol: 0mg

- Carbohydrates: 15g
- Fiber: 1g

Hot Apple Cider

Prep Time: 5 minutes

Cooking Time: 10 minutes

Serving Size: 1 cup

Ingredients:

- 4 cups unsweetened apple juice (low potassium)
- 1 cinnamon stick
- 4 cloves
- 1 orange, thinly sliced
- 1 tablespoon lemon juice

Instructions:

1. Combine apple juice, cinnamon stick, cloves, and orange slices in a large pot.
2. Bring to a simmer over medium heat. Reduce heat to low and continue simmering for 10 minutes to infuse the flavors.
3. Remove from heat and stir in lemon juice.
4. Strain the mixture to remove solids before serving.
5. Serve the cider hot.

Nutritional Information (per serving):

- Calories: 120
- Protein: 0g
- Sodium: 10mg
- Potassium: 280mg
- Total Fat: 0g
- Saturated Fat: 0g

- Cholesterol: 0mg
- Carbohydrates: 30g
- Fiber: 0.5g

Hot Holiday Cider (Low Sugar)

Prep Time: 5 minutes

Cooking Time: 10 minutes

Serving Size: 1 cup

Ingredients:

- 4 cups unsweetened apple juice (low potassium)
- 2 cinnamon sticks
- 1/2 teaspoon allspice
- 1/2 teaspoon nutmeg
- Orange peel from 1 orange
- Stevia (or another sugar substitute) to taste

Instructions:

1. In a large pot, combine the apple juice, cinnamon sticks, allspice, nutmeg, and orange peel.
2. Heat over medium until the mixture reaches a simmer, then reduce heat to low. Simmer for 10 minutes.
3. Sweeten with stevia to taste.
4. Strain and serve hot.

Nutritional Information (per serving):

- Calories: 30 (varies with sweetener)
- Protein: 0g
- Sodium: 5mg
- Potassium: 280mg
- Total Fat: 0g
- Saturated Fat: 0g

- Cholesterol: 0mg
- Carbohydrates: 7g (varies with sweetener)
- Fiber: 0.5g

Lemon Cooler

Prep Time: 5 minutes

Cooking Time: 0 minutes

Serving Size: 1 cup

Ingredients:

- 1 cup cold water
- Juice of 1 lemon
- 1 teaspoon honey (optional, adjust based on dietary needs)
- Ice cubes
- Fresh mint leaves for garnish

Instructions:

1. In a glass, combine the cold water and lemon juice.
2. Sweeten with honey if desired, and stir until well mixed.
3. Add ice cubes to the glass.
4. Garnish with fresh mint leaves.
5. Serve immediately for a refreshing drink.

Nutritional Information (per serving):

- Calories: 15 (varies with honey)
- Protein: 0g
- Sodium: 0mg
- Potassium: 50mg
- Total Fat: 0g
- Saturated Fat: 0g
- Cholesterol: 0mg

- Carbohydrates: 5g (varies with honey)
- Fiber: 0g

Lemon Smoothie

Prep Time: 5 minutes

Cooking Time: 0 minutes

Serving Size: 1 cup

Ingredients:

- 1 cup unsweetened almond milk
- Juice of 1 lemon
- 1/2 banana, frozen
- 1 tablespoon chia seeds
- 1 teaspoon honey (optional, adjust based on dietary needs)
- Ice cubes

Instructions:

1. Place almond milk, lemon juice, frozen banana, chia seeds, and honey (if using) into a blender.
2. Blend until smooth.
3. Add ice cubes and blend again to reach the desired consistency.
4. Serve immediately.

Nutritional Information (per serving):

- Calories: 150
- Protein: 3g
- Sodium: 60mg
- Potassium: 200mg
- Total Fat: 4.5g
- Saturated Fat: 0g
- Cholesterol: 0mg
- Carbohydrates: 25g
- Fiber: 4g

Lemonade Cranberry Lime Protein Drink

Prep Time: 5 minutes

Cooking Time: 0 minutes

Serving Size: 1 cup

Ingredients:

- 1 cup low-sugar lemonade
- 1/4 cup unsweetened cranberry juice
- Juice of 1 lime
- 1 scoop unflavored whey protein powder (low in potassium and phosphorus)
- Ice cubes

Instructions:

1. In a blender, combine lemonade, cranberry juice, lime juice, and protein powder.
2. Blend until smooth.
3. Add ice cubes and blend again until the drink is cold and frothy.
4. Serve immediately in a chilled glass.

Nutritional Information (per serving):

- Calories: 120
- Protein: 20g
- Sodium: 50mg
- Potassium: 150mg
- Total Fat: 0.5g
- Saturated Fat: 0g
- Cholesterol: 30mg
- Carbohydrates: 8g
- Fiber: 0g

30-DAY MEAL PLAN

Day 1

- **Breakfast:** Banana Oat Shake
- **Lunch:** Apple Rice Salad
- **Dinner:** Moroccan Couscous
- **Dessert:** Baked Shrimp Rolls

Day 2

- **Breakfast:** Berrylicious Smoothie
- **Lunch:** Beef Barley Soup
- **Dinner:** Grilled Vegetables
- **Dessert:** Brown Sugar Apple Dip

Day 3

- **Breakfast:** Blueberry Lemon Pound Cake
- **Lunch:** Chicken and Dumplings
- **Dinner:** Apple Almond Galette
- **Snack:** Lemon Pepper Hummus

Day 4

- **Breakfast:** Lemon-Blueberry Corn Muffins
- **Lunch:** Creamy Tuna Twist
- **Dinner:** Bolognese with Rice Noodles
- **Dessert:** Buffalo Wings

Day 5

- **Breakfast:** Pumpkin Cream Cheese Muffins
- **Lunch:** Chinese Chicken Salad
- **Dinner:** Roasted Asparagus and Wild Mushroom Stew
- **Dessert:** Cereal Snack Mix with Salt-free Seasoning

Day 6

- **Breakfast:** Apple Puffs
- **Lunch:** Cider Cream Chicken
- **Dinner:** Creamy Curry Rice & Apple Salad
- **Snack:** Garlic Oyster Crackers

Day 7

- **Breakfast:** Bran Breakfast Bars
- **Lunch:** Curry Chicken Salad
- **Dinner:** Balsamic Marinated Mushrooms
- **Dessert:** Chicken Nuggets with Honey Mustard Dipping Sauce

Day 8

- **Breakfast:** Blueberry Oatmeal
- **Lunch:** Lemon Curry Chicken Salad
- **Dinner:** Blueberry Lemon Pound Cake
- **Snack:** Pickled Okra

Day 9

- **Breakfast:** Turkey Bacon, Egg, and Cheese Deviled Eggs
- **Lunch:** Grilled Vegetable Pasta Salad
- **Dinner:** Mexican Antojitos
- **Dessert:** Barbecue Meatballs

Day 10

- **Breakfast:** Chicken and Zucchini Quiche
- **Lunch:** Cowboy Caviar Bean and Rice Salad
- **Dinner:** Apple Cranberry Walnut Salad
- **Dessert:** Buffalo Chicken Dip

Day 11

- **Breakfast:** Banana-Apple Smoothie
- **Lunch:** Kohlrabi Soup
- **Dinner:** Grilled Vegetables with Herbed Vinaigrette
- **Snack:** Crispy-Crunch Snack Bars

Day 12

- **Breakfast:** Pumpkin Pancakes
- **Lunch:** Irish Baked Potato Soup
- **Dinner:** Favorite Cranberry Salad
- **Dessert:** Brie and Cranberry Chutney

Day 13

- **Breakfast:** Fruit Crisp
- **Lunch:** Lentil Meatballs or Patties
- **Dinner:** Apple Spice Cake
- **Snack:** Falafel

Day 14

- **Breakfast:** Grilled Low-Salt Flatbread
- **Lunch:** Chicken and Corn Chowder
- **Dinner:** Gelatin Beet Salad
- **Dessert:** Flour Tortilla Chips

Day 15

- **Breakfast:** Love Your Kidneys Breakfast Cereal
- **Lunch:** Canned Fish Tacos
- **Dinner:** Healthy Chicken Nuggets
- **Snack:** Raspberry Wings

Day 16

- **Breakfast:** Banana-Apple Smoothie
- **Lunch:** Chicken N' Orange Salad Sandwich
- **Dinner:** Moroccan Couscous
- **Dessert:** Flour Tortilla Chips

Day 17

- **Breakfast:** Pumpkin Cream Cheese Muffins
- **Lunch:** Canned Fish Tacos
- **Dinner:** Bolognese with Rice Noodles
- **Dessert:** Raspberry Wings

Day 18

- **Breakfast:** Blueberry Lemon Pound Cake
- **Lunch:** Chicken and Dumplings
- **Dinner:** Creamy Curry Rice & Apple Salad
- **Dessert:** Garlic Oyster Crackers

Day 19

- **Breakfast:** Blueberry Squares
- **Lunch:** Beef Barley Soup
- **Dinner:** Grilled Vegetables
- **Dessert:** Baked Shrimp Rolls

Day 20

- **Breakfast:** Bran Breakfast Bars
- **Lunch:** Cowboy Caviar Bean and Rice Salad
- **Dinner:** Roasted Asparagus and Wild Mushroom Stew
- **Dessert:** Barbecue Meatballs

Day 21

- **Breakfast:** Lemon-Blueberry Corn Muffins
- **Lunch:** Curry Chicken Salad
- **Dinner:** Apple Almond Galette
- **Dessert:** Brie and Cranberry Chutney

Day 22

- **Breakfast:** Peanut Butter Oatmeal

- **Lunch:** Creamy Tuna Twist
- **Dinner:** Balsamic Marinated Mushrooms
- **Dessert:** Brown Sugar Apple Dip

Day 23

- **Breakfast:** Pumpkin Pancakes
- **Lunch:** Herb Breaded Chicken
- **Dinner:** Apple Sage Stuffing
- **Dessert:** Buffalo Chicken Dip

Day 24

- **Breakfast:** Turkey Bacon, Egg, and Cheese Deviled Eggs
- **Lunch:** Lemon Curry Chicken Salad
- **Dinner:** Favorite Cranberry Salad
- **Dessert:** Buffalo Wings

Day 25

- **Breakfast:** Love Your Kidneys Breakfast Cereal
- **Lunch:** Lentil Meatballs or Patties
- **Dinner:** Apple Spice Cake
- **Dessert:** Cereal Snack Mix with Salt-free Seasoning

Day 26

- **Breakfast:** Grilled Low-Salt Flatbread
- **Lunch:** Kohlrabi Soup
- **Dinner:** Gelatin Beet Salad

- **Dessert:** Chicken Nuggets with Honey Mustard Dipping Sauce

Day 27

- **Breakfast:** Fruit Crisp
- **Lunch:** Irish Baked Potato Soup
- **Dinner:** Healthy Chicken Nuggets
- **Dessert:** Chicken Parmesan Meatballs

Day 28

- **Breakfast:** Cranberry Ginger Apricot Chutney
- **Lunch:** Grilled Vegetable Pasta Salad
- **Dinner:** Grilled Vegetables with Herbed Vinaigrette
- **Dessert:** Chicken Pepper Bacon Wraps

Day 29

- **Breakfast:** Chicken and Zucchini Quiche
- **Lunch:** Green Tomatoes with Goat Cheese
- **Dinner:** Mexican Antojitos
- **Dessert:** Crispy-Crunch Snack Bars

Day 30

- **Breakfast:** Berrylicious Smoothie
- **Lunch:** Bow-Tie Pasta Salad
- **Dinner:** Baked Potato Soup
- **Dessert:** Falafel

BONUS CHAPTER: INTERACTIVE TOOLS

Daily Food and Fluid Intake Diary

Date: _____________________

Name: _____________________

Breakfast

Time	Food Item	Portion Size	Sodium (mg)	Potassium (mg)	Phosphorus (mg)	Protein (g)	Fluids (ml)

Morning Snack

Time	Food Item	Portion Size	Sodium (mg)	Potassium (mg)	Phosphorus (mg)	Protein (g)	Fluids (ml)

Lunch

Time	Food Item	Portion Size	Sodium (mg)	Potassium (mg)	Phosphorus (mg)	Protein (g)	Fluids (ml)

Afternoon Snack

Time	Food Item	Portion Size	Sodium (mg)	Potassium (mg)	Phosphorus (mg)	Protein (g)	Fluids (ml)

Dinner

Time	Food Item	Portion Size	Sodium (mg)	Potassium (mg)	Phosphorus (mg)	Protein (g)	Fluids (ml)

Evening Snack

Time	Food Item	Portion Size	Sodium (mg)	Potassium (mg)	Phosphorus (mg)	Protein (g)	Fluids (ml)

Total Daily Intake

- **Sodium (mg):**
- **Potassium (mg):**
- **Phosphorus (mg):**
- **Protein (g):**
- **Fluids (ml):**

Notes/Observations:

____

____

____

____

____

Medication Management Worksheet

Patient Name: _______________________________________

Date: _____________________

Instructions: Please fill out this worksheet daily. List all medications, including prescription drugs, over-the-counter medications, and any supplements you are taking. Include the reason for each medication, the dosage, and the time of day it should be taken, and any special instructions. Remember to bring this sheet to your healthcare appointments.

Time of Day	Medication Name	Dosage (mg, mL, etc.)	Reason for Medication	Special Instructions	Taken (✓)
Morning					
Noon					
Evening					
Night					

Notes/Comments:

____

____

____

____

Doctor's Name: _______________________________________

Doctor's Contact Information: _______________________________________

Pharmacy Contact Information: _______________________________________

Next Appointment: Date: ____________ Time: ___________

Instructions for Use:

- **Medication Name:** Write the name of the medication.
- **Dosage:** Include the amount of medication prescribed.
- **Reason for Medication:** Briefly describe why you are taking this medication.
- **Special Instructions:** Note any specific instructions such as "take with food" or "avoid sunlight."
- **Taken (✓):** Mark with a check once the medication has been taken.

Blood Pressure Log

Patient Name: ____

Month/Year: ____

Instructions: Record your blood pressure readings twice a day, preferably at the same times each day (e.g., morning and evening). Note any factors that might have influenced your reading, such as stress, exercise, or changes in medication.

Date	Time of Day	Systolic (mm Hg)	Diastolic (mm Hg)	Heart Rate (beats per minute)	Notes (Medication changes, dietary factors, exercise, stress, etc.)
	Morning				
	Evening				
	Morning				
	Evening				
	Morning				
	Evening				
	Morning				
	Evening				
	Morning				
	Evening				

Weekly Summary / Observations:

Week Ending (Date)	Average Morning Systolic	Average Morning Diastolic	Average Evening Systolic	Average Evening Diastolic	Overall Observations

Notes / Comments:

____

____

____

____

____

____

Lab Test Tracker

Patient Name: _______________________________________

Date of Birth: _______________________________________

Physician's Name: _______________________________________

Last Updated: _______________________________________

Key Indicators

Date	Glomerular Filtration Rate (GFR)	Creatinine (mg/dL)	Blood Urea Nitrogen (BUN) (mg/dL)	Potassium (K+) (mmol/L)	Phosphorus (P) (mg/dL)	Calcium (Ca2+) (mg/dL)	Hemoglobin (g/dL)	Albumin (g/dL)

Additional Tests

Date	Test Name	Result	Reference Range	Notes

Physician's Notes

- **[Date YYYY-MM-DD]:**
    - Note 1: ____
    - Note 2: ____
- **[Date YYYY-MM-DD]:**
    - Note 1: ____
    - Note 2: ____

Symptom Tracker

Patient Name: ___________________________________

Date of Birth: ___________________________________

Physician's Name: ___________________________________

Last Updated: ___________________________________

Daily Symptom Log

Date	Time	Symptom Description	Severity (1-10)	Duration	Action Taken (Medication/Rest/Other)	Notes
		Example: Swelling in ankles	5	2 hours	Elevated feet, rested	

Weekly Summary & Observations

Week of [Start Date] - [End Date]:

- **General Well-being:**
    - Overall mood:

    ____

    - Energy levels:

    ____

- **Dietary Notes:**
    - Changes in appetite: _______________________________________
    - Specific cravings or aversions: _______________________________
- **Physical Activity:**
    - Types of activities: _______________________________________
    - Any difficulty during exercise: _______________________________
- **Other Observations:**

-
-

Notes for Next Physician Visit

1.
2.
3.

Exercise Log

Patient Name: ____

Date of Birth: ____

Physician's Name: ____

Last Updated: ____

Weekly Exercise Schedule

Date	Type of Exercise	Duration	Intensity Level	Notes on How I Felt Before, During, and After Exercise
YYYY-MM-DD	Example: Walking	30 minutes	Low	Felt energetic before, moderate tiredness during, refreshed after

Exercise Goals

- **Short-term Goal:** ____
- **Long-term Goal:** ____

Weekly Reflections and Adjustments

- **[Week Starting YYYY-MM-DD]:**
    - Achievements:

      ____

    - Challenges:

      ____

    - Adjustments for Next Week: ____

Appointment and Questions Tracker

Patient Name: ____

Date of Birth: ____

Primary Care Physician: ______________________________

Nephrologist: ____

Other Specialists: _________________________________

Upcoming Appointments

Date	Time	Doctor/Specialist	Location	Purpose of Visit	Questions/Concerns
YYYY-MM-DD	HH:MM	Example: Dr. Smith, Nephrologist	Example: City Medical Center, Room 502	Routine check-up	1. Update on kidney function?

Past Appointments Summary

Date	Doctor/Specialist	Key Takeaways & Recommendations
YYYY-MM-DD	Example: Dr. Smith, Nephrologist	Discussed current kidney function. Suggested reducing sodium intake.

Medication Adjustments

Date	Medication	Adjustment (e.g., dosage change, new medication)	Reason
YYYY-MM-DD	Example: Lisinopril	Reduced to 10mg from 20mg	Lower blood pressure to target range

Notes for Next Visit

- **[Date YYYY-MM-DD]:**
  - Question 1:

    ____
  - Question 2:

    ____
  - Concerns:

    ____

Mood and Well-being Journal

Patient Name: ___________________________________

Date of Birth: ___________________________________

Physician's Name: ___________________________________

Last Updated: ___________________________________

Daily Mood Log

Date	Mood (1-10)	Stress Level (1-10)	Sleep Quality (1-10)	Energy Level (1-10)	General Well-being Notes
YYYY-MM-DD					Example: Felt anxious in the morning, improved after a walk. Good energy levels in the afternoon.

Weekly Reflection

Week of [Start Date] - [End Date]:

- **Overall Mood Summary:**
  - _______________________________________

- **What improved my mood:**
  - _______________________________________

- **What worsened my mood:**

-
- **Goals for Next Week:**
    - Focus more on relaxation techniques.
    - Increase physical activity to boost mood and energy.

Emotional Health Strategies

- **Relaxation Techniques Tried:**
    - Meditation, Deep Breathing, etc.

- **Physical Activities:**
    - Walks, Yoga, etc.

- **Social Interactions:**
    - Calls with family/friends, Support group meetings, etc.

Notes for Next Physician or Therapist Visit

- **Questions/Concerns:**
    1.
    2.

Emergency Contact Sheet

Patient Name: ___________________________________

Date of Birth: ___________________________________

Primary Care Physician: ___________________________

Nephrologist: ___________________________________

Other Specialists: ________________________________

Personal Information

- **Address:** ____
- **Phone Number:** _______________________________________
- **Blood Type:** ____
- **Allergies:** ____
- **Current Medications:** _________________________________

Emergency Contacts

Name	Relationship	Primary Phone	Secondary Phone	Email Address
Example: Jane Doe	Daughter	(555) 123-4567	(555) 765-4321	jane.doe@email.com

Healthcare Providers

Provider Name	Specialty	Phone Number	Email Address	Office Address
Example: Dr. Smith	Nephrologist	(555) 234-5678	drsmith@medicalcenter.com	123 Health St, City, State

			164	

Insurance Information

- **Provider:** ____
- **Member ID:** ____
- **Group Number:** ____
- **Contact Number:** ____

Additional Notes

____

____

____

____

____

CONCLUSION

In this comprehensive journey through the culinary landscape tailored for seniors with Stage 4 Kidney Disease, we've explored a variety of recipes designed to nourish the body while satisfying the palate. From the comforting warmth of Pumpkin Pancakes to the delightful zest of Lemon-Blueberry Corn Muffins, each recipe has been crafted with the dual goals of health and flavor in mind. These dishes not only cater to specific dietary needs but also embrace the joy of eating, proving that a kidney-friendly diet can be both delicious and diverse.

Understanding the importance of dietary management in kidney disease, we delved into the principles of a heart-healthy diet, emphasizing the roles of fiber and antioxidants, and the necessity of balancing nutrients such as potassium, phosphorus, and sodium. The recipes provided serve as a testament to the possibility of enjoying a rich tapestry of flavors while adhering to dietary restrictions, offering a beacon of hope and a source of inspiration for those navigating the complexities of kidney disease.

The journey through meal planning and preparation has underscored the significance of being informed and proactive about dietary choices. By highlighting strategies for eating well both at home and outside, we've aimed to empower individuals with the knowledge and confidence needed to make healthful food choices in any setting. The detailed instructions and nutritional information accompanying each recipe are designed to demystify the process of cooking for kidney health, making it accessible to everyone, regardless of their culinary expertise.

Moreover, this exploration has been more than just about food; it's been a journey of discovery, resilience, and adaptation. It reflects a deeper understanding of how diet can play a pivotal role in managing chronic conditions and the impact of thoughtful food choices on overall well-being. The recipes and strategies shared here are not just guidelines but stepping stones to a healthier, more vibrant life, even in the face of kidney disease.

As we conclude this culinary adventure, it's important to remember that each individual's journey is unique, and what works for one person may not work for another. Therefore, collaboration with healthcare professionals, including dietitians and nephrologists, is crucial to tailor dietary plans to meet personal health needs and preferences. This book is intended to be a resource, a companion in the kitchen, and a source of inspiration, but it is by no means a substitute for professional medical advice.

To our dear readers, thank you for embarking on this journey with us. Your health, joy, and satisfaction have been our guiding lights in crafting this collection of recipes and insights. We hope that these pages have provided you with valuable tools and knowledge to navigate your dietary needs with confidence and creativity. Your resilience and commitment to your health journey are truly commendable, and we are honored to have been a part of it.

As you continue to explore the flavors and possibilities within these pages, we invite you to share your experiences, discoveries, and feedback. If this book has found a place in your kitchen and your heart, we would be grateful for an honest review on Amazon. Your thoughts and insights not only help us improve but also serve as a beacon for others navigating similar paths, guiding them toward a healthier, more flavorful future.

Thank you for allowing us to be a part of your culinary adventure. Here's to many more delicious and healthful meals ahead.

MEAL PLANNER

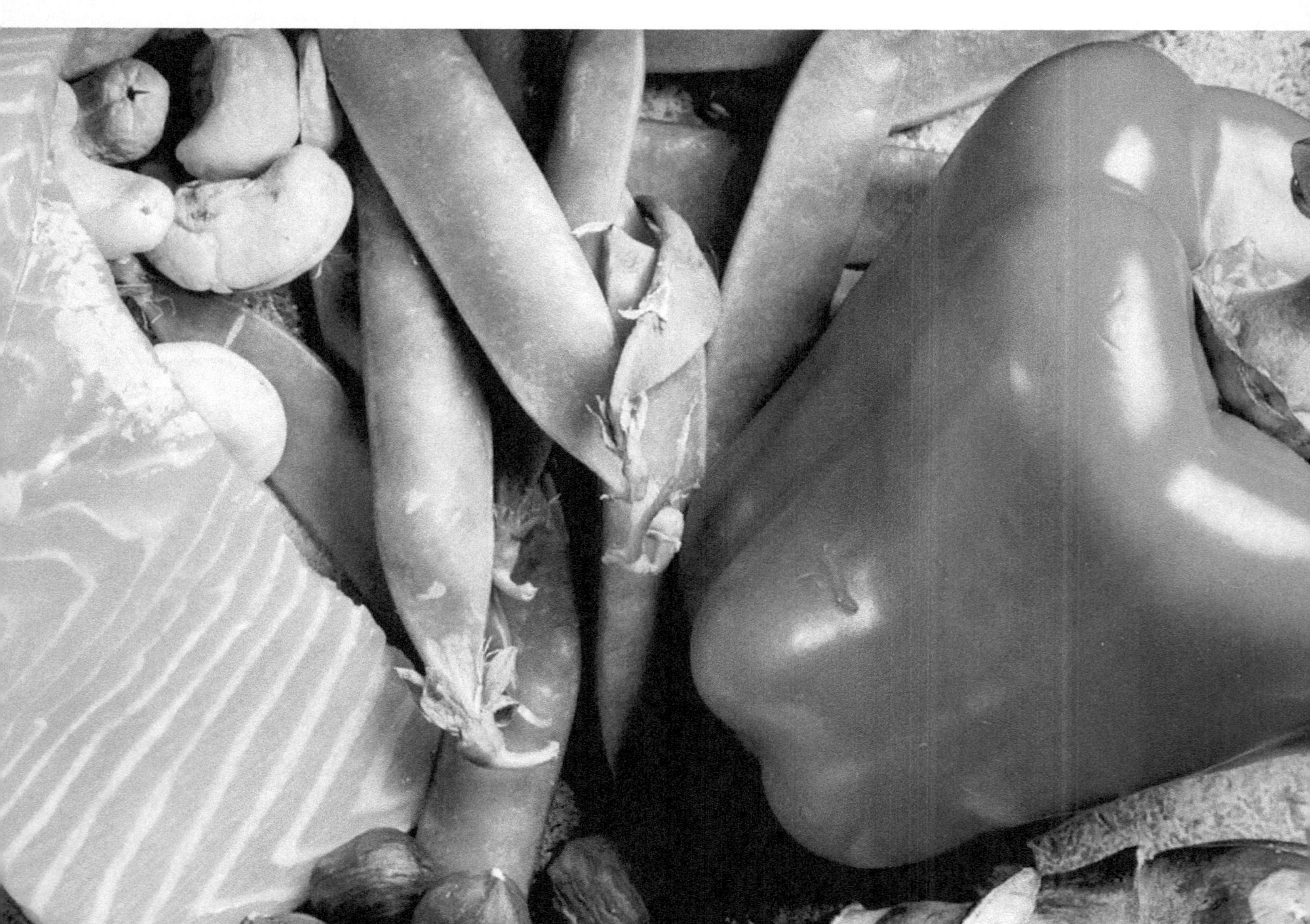

Weekly Meal Planner

Grocery List

	Breakfast	Lunch	Dinner	Snacks
mon				
tue				
wed				
thu				
fri				
sat				
sun				

Weekly Meal Planner

Grocery List

	Breakfast	Lunch	Dinner	Snacks
mon				
tue				
wed				
thu				
fri				
sat				
sun				

Weekly Meal Planner

Grocery List

	Breakfast	Lunch	Dinner	Snacks
mon				
tue				
wed				
thu				
fri				
sat				
sun				

Weekly Meal Planner

Grocery List

	Breakfast	Lunch	Dinner	Snacks
mon				
tue				
wed				
thu				
fri				
sat				
sun				

Weekly Meal Planner

Grocery List

	Breakfast	Lunch	Dinner	Snacks
mon				
tue				
wed				
thu				
fri				
sat				
sun				

Weekly Meal Planner

Grocery List

	Breakfast	Lunch	Dinner	Snacks
mon				
tue				
wed				
thu				
fri				
sat				
sun				

Weekly Meal Planner

Grocery List

	Breakfast	Lunch	Dinner	Snacks
mon				
tue				
wed				
thu				
fri				
sat				
sun				

Weekly Meal Planner

Grocery List

	Breakfast	Lunch	Dinner	Snacks
mon				
tue				
wed				
thu				
fri				
sat				
sun				

Weekly Meal Planner

Grocery List

	Breakfast	Lunch	Dinner	Snacks
mon				
tue				
wed				
thu				
fri				
sat				
sun				

Weekly Meal Planner

Grocery List

	Breakfast	Lunch	Dinner	Snacks
mon				
tue				
wed				
thu				
fri				
sat				
sun